THE BREAST TEST BOOK

The Breast Test Book

A WOMAN'S GUIDE TO MAMMOGRAPHY AND BEYOND

Connie Jones, MD
MEDICAL DIRECTOR,
SOLIS MAMMOGRAPHY, ARIZONA

Michael N. Linver, MD, FACR, FSBI
DIRECTOR OF MAMMOGRAPHY,
X-RAY ASSOCIATES OF NEW MEXICO, PC (RETIRED)
CLINICAL PROFESSOR OF RADIOLOGY,
UNIVERSITY OF NEW MEXICO
DIRECTOR OF BREAST IMAGING BOOT CAMP TEACHING COURSES,
AMERICAN COLLEGE OF RADIOLOGY

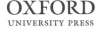

OXFORD
UNIVERSITY PRESS

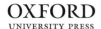

OXFORD
UNIVERSITY PRESS

Oxford University Press is a department of the University of Oxford. It furthers
the University's objective of excellence in research, scholarship, and education
by publishing worldwide. Oxford is a registered trade mark of Oxford University
Press in the UK and certain other countries.

Published in the United States of America by Oxford University Press
198 Madison Avenue, New York, NY 10016, United States of America.

Library of Congress Cataloging-in-Publication Data
Names: Jones, Connie (Connie Phillips), 1965–
Title: The breast test book : a woman's guide to mammography and beyond /
Connie Jones, MD, Medical Director, Solis Mammography, Arizona,
Medical Director of Breast Imaging, Abrazo Arrowhead Campus.
Description: New York, NY : Oxford University Press, [2017]
Identifiers: LCCN 2017033343 | ISBN 9780190677053 (paperback)
Subjects: LCSH: Breast—Cancer—Diagnosis. | Breast—Examination. |
BISAC: MEDICAL / Oncology. | MEDICAL / General.
Classification: LCC RC280.B8 J66 2017 | DDC 616.99/449075—dc23
LC record available at https://lccn.loc.gov/2017033343

This material is not intended to be, and should not be considered, a substitute for medical or other professional
advice. Treatment for the conditions described in this material is highly dependent on the individual
circumstances. And, while this material is designed to offer accurate information with respect to the subject
matter covered and to be current as of the time it was written, research and knowledge about medical and health
issues is constantly evolving and dose schedules for medications are being revised continually, with new side
effects recognized and accounted for regularly. Readers must therefore always check the product information
and clinical procedures with the most up-to-date published product information and data sheets provided by
the manufacturers and the most recent codes of conduct and safety regulation. The publisher and the authors
make no representations or warranties to readers, express or implied, as to the accuracy or completeness of this
material. Without limiting the foregoing, the publisher and the authors make no representations or warranties as
to the accuracy or efficacy of the drug dosages mentioned in the material. The authors and the publisher do not
accept, and expressly disclaim, any responsibility for any liability, loss or risk that may be claimed or incurred as a
consequence of the use and/or application of any of the contents of this material.

9 8 7 6 5 4 3 2 1

Printed by Sheridan Books, Inc., United States of America

This book is dedicated to the memory of my mother, Jacquelyn Phillips, who loved and supported me with every fiber of her being every day of her life. With the publication of this book, she will finally get the satisfaction of knowing that it is abundantly clear to all that a radiologist is a real medical doctor!

If there is a book you want to read but it has not been written yet, then you must write it.

TONI MORRISON

.

Contents

Foreword ix

Acknowledgments xi

PART I | FIRST THINGS FIRST

1. Breast Imaging: Until There Is a Cure: The Unknown Frontier in Women's Health 3

2. The Screening Mammogram Guidelines Controversy: What You Absolutely Must Know: Addressing the Elephant in the Room, and the Case for Tomosynthesis 11

PART II | THE WHO

3. You! How You Impact Your Care: Your Responsibilities and Information You Need to Know 23

4. The Breast Imaging Team: Radiologist, Technologists, and Navigator 32

5. The Rulers of Mammoland: MQSA, ACR, SBI, and the Other ABCs of Imaging 36

6. Your Referring Doctor: The Delicate Balance of the Referral-Consult Relationship 38

PART III | THE WHAT

7. The Tools of Breast Imaging: A Picture Is Worth a Thousand Words 43

PART IV | THE WHY

8. How It All Works: An Overview: A Bird's-Eye View of the Whole Process 53

9. How It All Works: The Screening Evaluation: Screening the Asymptomatic Population and Saving Lives 56

vii

10. *How It All Works: The Diagnostic Evaluation: Symptomatic Patients and the Journey to the Correct Diagnosis* 66

11. *Breast Urgent-cies: This Cannot Wait Until Tomorrow!* 111

12. *You Need a Biopsy—Don't Panic!: Image-Guided Needle Biopsy: A Remarkable Advance in Technology and Patient Care* 114

13. *You Do Not Have Breast Cancer: The Value of a Benign Evaluation* 127

14. *You Have Been Diagnosed With Breast Cancer: The Critical Role of Radiology in Treatment Planning and Follow-up* 139

PART V | OTHER CONSIDERATIONS

15. *Special Cases: Pregnancy, Lactation, Breast Implants, Lymphoproliferative Disorders and Male Breast Cancer* 151

16. *How Does Your Report Get to You and Your Doctor?: No News Is Not Necessarily Good News* 156

17. *Patients' Questions About the Imaging Evaluation: Learning More Can Save Your Life* 159

PART VI | BREAST IMAGING MEETS THE OUTSIDE WORLD

18. *Medicolegal Issues and Liability: Can Breast Imaging Survive the Liability Crisis?* 167

19. *Safety Issues in Mammography and Breast Imaging: Assessing the Risk-Benefit Ratio* 169

20. *The Breast Density Discussion: Information versus Notification* 173

GLOSSARY 1: TOPICS IN BREAST IMAGING: TERMINOLOGY 101 179
GLOSSARY 2: BREAST HEALTH VOCABULARY: QUICK REFERENCE, ALPHABETICAL 197
BIBLIOGRAPHY 209
INDEX 215

Foreword

IT IS WITH great pleasure and admiration that I write this foreword and serve as editor for Dr. Connie Jones' superb overview of mammography and related tests for breast cancer detection used in radiology. Dr. Jones brings a rare and complimentary combination of excellent training, extensive practical experience, and the skills to mold complex medical issues into an easily understandable narrative.

As a fellow radiologist who has practiced breast imaging as my specialty for 30 years primarily in a nonacademic setting, I appreciate Dr. Jones' ability to bring all the important issues surrounding the complicated and often controversial subjects we confront in breast imaging to light, including how a mammogram is performed and interpreted, when mammography should or should not be performed, what imaging tests are performed to supplement the mammogram and when they are applied, what happens when breast cancer is suspected on a mammogram, and what the next steps are if a cancer is found. She provides a lucid guide for women everywhere so that the true lifesaving value of breast imaging can be not only appreciated, but fully understood.

Dr. Jones fills a critical void in the medical world. For the first time, women have a friend and guide to take with them on their journey through the health care system in terms they can understand, a journey that may conclude by saving their lives.

I applaud Dr. Jones and thank her for taking time from her busy practice to present us with this marvelous medical gift. It is a gift that comes from the heart, out of her passion for her work and her compassion for the patients she serves. Bravo, Dr. Jones!

Michael N. Linver, MD, FACR, FSBI
Director of Mammography
X-Ray Associates of New Mexico, PC
Clinical Professor of Radiology
University of New Mexico
Director of Breast Imaging Boot Camp teaching courses
American College of Radiology

Acknowledgments

THE CONCEPT AND compilation of this book has been many years in the making. As a practicing physician for over 20 years I decided to write this book because I was frustrated by the many misconceptions my patients had about the breast imaging process and I was disheartened that I could never find an appropriate book to recommend to them. So, I decided to write this book—for them.

Firstly, I would like to acknowledge and sincerely thank the brilliant radiologists and researchers in the field of Breast Imaging. Their contribution has been paramount to the development of this book. And without their diligence and hard work there would be no such thing as Breast Radiology as a subspecialty. Their work is the basis for my knowledge of the subject matter in this book.

The content and conclusions derived in the book were developed over the many years of my medical practice as a *dedicated Breast Imaging Radiologist* in a community practice setting. So, while there are some citations the opinions in the text are mine based on years of experience and encounters with thousands of patients and referring physicians and assessing literally thousands of images. If I have failed to cite an appropriate source, I am truly sorry.

I am honored and very grateful to have the input and editorial assistance of Dr. Michael Linver for this book. He has been a superb mentor and a good friend. As an experienced Breast Radiologist and nationally and internationally recognized educator his experience and insight were invaluable to assuring that the material in the book was relevant and accurate. His contribution to the chapters on the screening controversy, dense breast discussion, medical legal and safety issues in mammography were invaluable. His wife Mina Jo (an amazing person in her own right) was also instrumental in giving me strategies to secure publication and market visibility. Mike and Mina Jo your support has been critical to the success of this endeavor. Thank you.

Special thanks goes to LuAnn Roberson, RN. She is an extraordinary nurse navigator by any measure only overshadowed by her integrity and strength of character as a human being. Like many experienced nurses she subtly (and not so subtly) taught this doctor a few things about patient care and interaction. Her presence as my professional partner and her involvement as a consultant adds a completeness to the patient care aspects of the book that would not be possible without her.

Many, many thanks go to the mammography technologists and ultrasound technologists that I have worked with over the years. You have taught me so much. Thank you for your support and friendship.

I am particularly grateful to two colleagues who took the time to painstakingly review several chapters in great detail and offered very useful suggestions and edits. The first is Dr. Eric Groskind a fellow breast imager who I have great respect for as a physician and as a person. The second is Dr. Victor Zannis, an accomplished and nationally known breast surgeon whose input on the clinical aspects of the book were invaluable.

Thanks goes to my partner Dr. Millicent Gentry who generously assisted me with citing references even though it was quite a tedious job. And thanks is also extended to Dr. Pablo Pritchard who provided expert review of the plastic surgery related portions of the book.

I am deeply indebted to my fellowship director, Dr. John "Chip" Coscia who trained me to be a "clinical breast imager," not just a reader of films. That style of practice has served me well and has given me great satisfaction and purpose in my work.

I have worked with many outstanding radiologists, but I would like to thank two who were uniquely special and significant in my career, Dr. Bonna Rogers-Neufeld and Dr. Lori Kunzelman. Ladies your passion and dedication to your work and to your patients was remarkable and was an inspiration to me. I am honored to have worked beside you both and I learned so much in the interaction.

Sincere thanks goes to Bobbie Smothers Jones and Debbie Phillips who served as my "test audience." These intelligent thoughtful women gave useful practical advice and editing that helped me tremendously.

I have been blessed in this life to have a wonderful family and friends (who are like family). It has made all the difference. Thank you all for being there.

Specifically, I am grateful for the support and assistance of my son, Yannick Jones. He has been there through the many iterations and stages of this work giving encouragement throughout the many years of this process. He is also the photographer for my author photo. Great Job, Yannick!

I would like to especially thank my husband, Rick Anglin, who has always believed in me and whose loving encouragement always came at the right moment. His consistency, integrity and strength give me comfort in this very uncertain world.

I would like to thank Mark Pate for providing some of the illustrations for the book.

Lastly, I would like to thank my senior editor Andrea Knobloch who believed in this work and without whom this book would not have come to fruition. She and her editorial assistant Allison Pratt provided expert guidance and kept me on track in the unfamiliar world of publishing. Additionally, the production and copyediting team were superb.

First Things First

1

Breast Imaging: Until There Is a Cure

THE UNKNOWN FRONTIER IN WOMEN'S HEALTH

"HI, THERE. HOW ARE YOU? I'm Dr. Jones. It's nice to meet you."

Tara, an attractive young mother of three, is sitting on the ultrasound table with the look of anxious anticipation on her face—the deer in the headlights expression. Sensing her anxiety, which is common among patients in this setting, I try to calm her fears while not falsely implying that everything is copacetic. I haven't had a chance to look at the area, and I need to be certain of the findings before I give her my final assessment.

I personalize my greeting by taking her hand and give her my "girl handshake"—a light handshake that is more like a handhold. I always found it calming when my mother comforted me in this way; it helped me to concentrate on what she was saying, and I felt safe in her care.

I tell Tara that "things are looking pretty good so far" but that I want to look at the area with the ultrasound before making a final recommendation. I tell her that I will discuss the findings with her after I have completed the evaluation.

Now at her side, I continue, "We called you back today because your screening mammogram showed three nodules in your left breast that were new compared with your prior studies., The purpose of the examination today is to further evaluate those areas."

After the ultrasound technologist had evaluated the areas of concern, we reviewed the images together on the computer screen in the reading room. Two of the nodules are clearly cysts. One nodule has a slightly different appearance, but it is also likely to be a cyst. However, this conclusion is not definitive from review of the static (photograph-like) images, and this is the area that I want to scrutinize in real time as the examination is being performed (much like viewing a movie scene on a television screen). As I take the ultrasound probe, apply the gel, and place the transducer on her breast, I can tell that

Tara is closely observing my face for any hint of an untoward expression—any expression that might imply that I think the area represents breast cancer. I continue to display a pleasant poker face.

My evaluation reveals a cyst with mobile debris. Great. "Wonderful news, Tara," I say. "All of the areas that were of initial concern are confirmed to be cysts. Cysts are not cancer, and we don't have to do anything about them unless they are causing you problems. There is no need for any further assessment or follow-up, and we will see you next year for your annual mammogram."

A nanosecond later, there is a great big smile on her face, and she releases an audible sigh of relief. Then, suddenly, her eyes begin to well, and she bursts into tears. "I'm so relieved! I thought for sure you were going to tell me that I had breast cancer!" The technologist hands her a tissue, and I put my hand on her leg to comfort her.

Still crying, she says, "I feel so embarrassed. I don't usually act like this. I didn't realize I was *this* worried about this until now." As it turns out, she had not been sleeping well since she received the notice 3 days ago to return for an additional diagnostic (problem-solving) evaluation. She had called her friend Cathy last night because Cathy had had a breast biopsy last year and Tara thought that she could perhaps offer some advice. However, she had wanted to spare her mother the worry and decided to wait until after the evaluation before talking to her.

Sound familiar? Tara is by no means unusual in her response to this situation. She is usually not an overly emotional person and certainly can hold her own in other arenas of life, but this situation just seems to hit close to home for some reason. She is only my second diagnostic patient of the day. There are 20 more scheduled.

Later in the morning, Susan presents to the breast center for a diagnostic evaluation. She is being recalled because of new calcifications in her right breast that were seen on a recent screening mammogram. I inform her that the calcifications are suspicious and that she needs a biopsy. I review the films with her and then call the report to her referring physician. Susan will return to our facility in 4 days and undergo a stereotactic needle biopsy.

Susan's calcifications are ultimately confirmed to be malignant: ductal carcinoma in situ (highlighted terms are defined in the Glossary). Fortunately, because she has been getting annual screenings, the cancer has been detected early. She has an early-stage and probably curable disease.

Sadly, on the other end of the spectrum, there is Betty, who has had such a fear of being diagnosed with cancer—you don't have cancer until a doctor *tells* you that you have cancer—that she has never even had a screening mammogram. She is now 53 years old. She has felt a lump in her right breast for more than a year. It is now breaking through the skin and has an overlying infection. She has been conscientiously packing the wound with gauze and applying cream for several months. Until now she has refused any imaging evaluation. However, because of the foul smell, her husband has insisted that she come in to have it evaluated. He accompanies her to the evaluation.

All of the appropriate imaging studies are performed and reveal a spiculated mass (i.e., having "fingers") that is attached to her chest wall muscle. There is obvious skin involvement. An axillary (armpit) lymph node appears enlarged as well. Because she is at high risk of not returning (because her ambivalence has kept her away this long), consent is obtained, and a needle biopsy is performed on the same day for tissue diagnosis.

The biopsy findings confirmed that Betty has advanced right breast cancer and that it has metastasized (i.e., spread) to her regional lymph nodes and distally (i.e., far away) to her bones. Her prognosis (i.e., long-term outcome) is poor.

Today, four patients are scheduled for image-guided needle breast biopsies. Two are performed with stereotactic (mammogram) guidance, one with ultrasound guidance, and one with magnetic resonance imaging (MRI) guidance.

Roberta is scheduled for the ultrasound-guided core needle biopsy. She will have a biopsy of a lump that her doctor noticed on a clinical breast examination during her routine checkup last week. Roberta is very nervous and tearful and has taken a valium in advance of the procedure to calm her nerves. She also has brought her pastor, her parents, and her husband to the appointment for emotional support. During the process of the biopsy, we talk about her two favorite subjects: Ryan, age 4, and Cole, age 18 months. The biopsy is successful, and I am able to gather a sufficient amount of tissue for analysis. Roberta requires much supportive care, but she is able to successfully complete the examination. Two days later, the final pathology report is available. It says she has a benign (i.e., noncancerous) tumor called a fibroadenoma.

At the start of the day, I evaluated and then dictated reports on 45 of the screening mammograms that were performed the previous day at our screening facility. I recalled four patients because of abnormalities that I detected, and these ladies will become the diagnostic patients for next week. The cycle continues.

None of the patients described here are real, but the scenarios certainly are. This could easily be a typical day at any breast imaging center, and I have lived this day or something like it many times. For most women, delving into the world of breast imaging is a leap into the abyss of the unknown, and this adds unnecessary anxiety to an already stressful situation. Couple this with the fear of breast cancer, and you can see how this is a situation where the emotions are high and the stakes are even higher. Author and comedian Carol Leifer once described her breast imaging experience on Real Time With Bill Maher as a "24-hour cancer scare, one of those horrible scenarios where *you* keep staying and *they* keep taking more films." Although Carol's findings were ultimately confirmed to be benign, her experience was a health care incident that changed her life.

The process of the breast imaging evaluation (e.g., mammography, ultrasound, breast MRI, breast biopsy) is adversely affected by anxious anticipation. A woman's fear is exacerbated by lack of knowledge of the process and of what to expect. The fact is that not every woman who goes in for a breast evaluation will have breast cancer.

In reality, the incidence of breast cancer in the United States (i.e., number of women in the population with the disease) is 125.3 cases per 100,000 women (i.e., 3 to 6 cases for every 1000 screening mammograms). An estimated 231,840 cases of primary breast cancer were diagnosed and roughly 40,290 breast cancer–related deaths occurred in 2015. These statistics are significant, and finding these cancers is critical to saving lives and improving outcomes for breast cancer patients. On the other hand, benign breast abnormalities and symptoms are quite common and impact many more lives than breast cancer does. Accurate diagnosis of these noncancerous conditions can alleviate much of the patient's anxiety, help her get treatment for her symptoms, and guide her doctor toward the correct plan of action.

Breast cancer is the most commonly diagnosed malignancy in women, and it is the second leading cause of cancer-related deaths in American women. Although cardiovascular-related deaths significantly outnumber breast cancer deaths, breast cancer is the most feared disease among American women. For this reason, there is a tremendous amount of anxiety about any breast-related symptoms and great trepidation about undergoing a screening mammogram. In addition to women of screening age, a significant percentage of women with breast-related symptoms require some sort of radiologic evaluation. Millions of radiologic studies are performed each year to evaluate these concerns and determine the presence or absence of disease, most notably breast cancer. Everything about a woman's experience in the radiology department is heightened because of this fear: "Will this be the day that I am told that I have breast cancer?"

Great strides have been made in an effort to heighten public awareness of breast cancer, with the emphasis on early detection using mammography, which is the key to decreasing mortality rates due to the disease. Although much has been written about breast cancer and current treatments, very little has been published about the actual process of diagnosing or excluding the disease. As a result of the tremendous advances and discoveries in the medical specialty of radiology, we now have myriad tools to use in the investigation process. For the radiologist, the basic question when assessing a screening or diagnostic study is whether there is a finding on the image that shows possible evidence (i.e., it is on the list of things to consider) or probable evidence (i.e., it is the likely thing to consider) of cancer. Standard protocols have been established based on research and experience that help to yield the most accurate results.

Early in my career, I began referring to the breast-centric environment in which I work as *Mammoland* because it is uniquely different from that of any other subspecialty. During its evolution, radiologists not working in breast imaging did not always fully appreciate its unique concerns, and referring doctors interpreted patient contact as undermining their authority: Since when do radiologists *talk* to patients? Mammoland is a fitting name because breast imaging is a combination of two worlds: traditional radiology and clinical medicine. It truly is a land of its own. Breast imaging is a blend of the imaging advances in radiology with the clinical knowledge and patient contact of traditional primary care medicine.

At this point, you may be asking yourself, what exactly is breast imaging? Breast imaging is a subspecialty of the field of radiology that is focused on the assessment of breast conditions using imaging techniques. Radiology, including breast imaging, is a consult specialty that provides assistance to other physicians in the care of their patients by supervising the performance of and providing expert assessment of imaging procedures. This subspecialty field uses various images or pictures to visualize the breast parenchyma (i.e., tissue). Based on known standards of appearance and other characteristics, the breast imaging radiologist can determine the presence or absence of disease or abnormality.

A certain subset of radiologic techniques can be used to diagnose and treat conditions. Within the specialty of breast imaging, numerous modalities are used to evaluate the breast, each providing a different way to see within the breast tissue. The best known tool in breast imaging is the mammogram, which is performed with the use of radiation or x-rays. Mammography is the only modality that has been proven to decrease mortality (i.e., death) associated with breast cancer. This is the consequence of early detection, which allows the possibility of earlier treatment, thereby increasing the likelihood of a favorable outcome (i.e., not dying of breast cancer). Mortality rates for breast cancer have steadily decreased since 1990, when screening mammography became a standard recommendation in the United States.

Other breast imaging studies include breast ultrasound or sonography (which uses sound waves), breast MRI, tomosynthesis (i.e., multiple, thin-section mammograms), contrast mammography, and breast-specific gamma imaging (i.e., molecular imaging looking at cell activity). All of these visualization methods assist in the evaluation of the breast tissue and breast-related symptoms to determine the presence or absence of breast cancer. Radiologists also use these modalities to guide them in the performance of various types of needle biopsies and in the treatment of certain conditions.

Women's advocacy (most notably by the Susan G. Komen Foundation) has had a tremendous impact on the specialty of breast imaging by increasing public awareness about breast cancer as well as pushing the medical community to focus more attention on the topic by sometimes critically pointing out our shortcomings. The last 20 years have seen an exponential advance in development and knowledge in the realm of breast imaging. The ground-breaking screening trials by Tabár and colleagues in Sweden proved the efficacy of screening mammograms in decreasing breast cancer deaths. Ecklund and coworkers developed significant improvements in the technical performance of mammograms that have allowed the tissue to be better evaluated and more tissue to be visualized on the image: If the cancer is not seen on the films, there is no chance of detecting it.

The work of Pisano and associates added digital mammography to the arsenal by proving its efficacy and usefulness in a large multisite study (DMIST). Breast ultrasound has become a standard test for evaluating breast abnormalities, adding valuable data and increasing the accuracy of the imaging evaluation, as demonstrated by Stavros.

The American Cancer Society recommends breast MRI in certain screening populations based on a large multisite research trial (ACRINN), and MRI is an invaluable problem-solving tool in breast cancer cases, thanks in great part to the dedicated work of Berg and Morris and their coworkers. Parker and colleagues developed needle biopsy techniques using image guidance (e.g., mammography, ultrasound, MRI) and this has now become the first-line procedure for tissue diagnosis in most patients. Because of Kopans, Sickles, and Linver and their associates, comprehensive education has contributed to better training of residents and practicing radiologists, increasing the quality of their assessments.

The introduction of tomosynthesis (i.e., three-dimensional mammography) has been a significant game changer. It improves our ability to find more cancers, especially small invasive cancers, while decreasing recall rates by 30% or more. The work of Rose and colleagues validates its use outside the academic environment—that is, in the community setting, where most U.S. breast imaging is performed. All of these advances allow radiologists to more reliably differentiate benign from malignant disease, find early-stage disease, and make the diagnosis before surgery so that the patient can participate in the treatment and the surgeon can appropriately plan the surgery.

Forty years ago, it would not have been unusual for a woman to have a surgical biopsy and, if cancer were found, to wake up from the anesthesia without a breast—a decision made solely by her surgeon. As significant are the many women who have multiple breast scars as a result of having surgery after surgery after surgery (i.e., "patchwork breast"), or prophylactic mastectomy for *normal* lumpy breasts, as a result of the very limited tools available to evaluate breast abnormalities at the time. As a direct result of technologic advances and cutting-edge research, there are a greater number of tests, more sensitive tests, less invasive methods of biopsy, more data on which to base decision making, and more efficient and accurate methods of approaching breast care. We have come a long way.

Unique to the breast radiologist is the coupling of clinical proficiency in assessing symptoms and physical findings with skilled interpretation of imaging studies. This combination provides the most accurate assessment of breast-related problems. Based on training and experience, the radiologist is in a unique position to determine the type and frequency of examinations needed to address the clinical question. Radiologists are the only physicians sufficiently trained and skilled for this task. However, most people do not know that the radiologist is a medical doctor (M.D.) or that it is the radiologist, not their primary physician, who interprets their films. Other physicians may look at the films, but the radiologist interprets them based on years of training and application. The role of radiology in breast cancer detection and breast health has been largely unnoticed by the general public.

As a woman, I know that patients with a breast-related problem are eager to obtain information, but this pursuit can have vastly different outcomes depending on which sources are consulted. Those who are computer savvy can surf the web, and there are some good online sites (see the Resources section at the back of the book). Alternatively, women can get pamphlets from their local mammography facility or find an article in a woman's magazine. Most will call their best girlfriend or even their second cousin's roommate's mother (who had a similar problem last year) to get some sense of what their symptoms really mean and to gather advice about what to do next. Although friends and acquaintances are well intentioned, they are usually uninformed and give advice based on perceptions that may have little to do with a woman's particular situation. Although any or all of these things may be done, the quest is rarely satisfying or endowed with enough information to provide knowledgeable navigation through the process. Before her biopsy, one woman told me, "I looked online last night. I shouldn't have." She could not determine from her search which disease process applied to her, and as a result she was even more nervous about her possible outcome.

The goal of this book is to explain in understandable lay language the process of the breast imaging evaluation so that women who become patients can have a clearer idea of what to expect, making the process less emotionally charged and allowing full cooperation in their own care. In the event that the final diagnosis is cancer, there is an even greater benefit because the process of getting to the diagnosis is understood by you, the patient. I sometimes encounter women on the day of their breast cancer surgery who have little or no understanding of the reasoning behind the requested radiologic examination or procedure that is about to be performed.

The Breast Test Book can help women to incorporate this information into the whole scheme of their management, thereby increasing their confidence in the treatment plans. The book can familiarize readers with the mammogram and other imaging processes and provide helpful insights so that they can be more informed (and hopefully calmer) participants in their breast health care.

Why is *The Breast Test Book* being offered now? I have found that many books offering advice related to the topic of breast health are primarily about breast cancer. These books, usually written by surgeons and oncologists (i.e., cancer doctors), are about cancer, the worst outcome of a breast imaging evaluation. The discussion usually starts with the diagnosis of a malignant disease. Although these books are necessary and extremely useful for women who have been diagnosed with breast cancer, they leave out the millions of women seen in radiology departments each year who do not end up having cancer. Benign breast abnormalities and symptoms are considerably more common and impact many more lives than breast cancer does. Until recently, the field of radiology has allowed other specialties to present our position, usually with less than optimal effectiveness.

As a breast imaging radiologist practicing daily on the front lines of breast care in a busy community setting, I see in my patients every day the mental and emotional trauma that results from not having such a resource. Indeed, I have searched and been unable to find a suitable resource on the market to offer my patients. This book reflects my daily encounters with the needs of various doctors and their patients, both groups seeking clarification and direction. The information in this book is practical and can guide patients and their physicians seamlessly through the evaluation process while giving helpful hints in plain English about factors that assist with or detract from the process.

The book can assist patients in their journey into the world of mammography and breast imaging. The material is based on the solid fundamentals of current scientific research, established practice standards, and the many years of practical experience accumulated by a fellowship-trained, dedicated breast radiologist, the physician best trained to discuss the particulars of the breast imaging evaluation.

Readers will learn how the radiologist, a physician imaging expert, in his or her largely behind the scenes evaluation, often makes the most critical decisions and has the most impact on patient care. How does a woman's breast history impact the interpretation of her examination? Who gets screening mammography, and at what age should it begin? What is the difference between screening and diagnostic mammograms? What symptoms warrant a diagnostic (i.e., directed problem-solving) evaluation? When is ultrasound or MRI used? What characteristics determine whether a lesion is suspicious for cancer? Which lesions require biopsy? When should a needle biopsy be performed instead of surgical biopsy? Do implants affect the ability to detect cancer? If breast cancer is present, can imaging studies determine whether the patient is a candidate for lumpectomy or needs a mastectomy? Are there any breast imaging emergencies? These types of questions stir up much interest and even more emotion.

My hope is that the information in the book will debunk the myths, clarify misinformation, and provide clear, relevant, and easy to understand information on the subject matter. This book is not a research text or a journal article aimed at physicians but a common-sense guide for women who want to participate more fully in their own breast health. I like the way professor Bobbie Smothers Jones put it: "You are discussing exactly what I need to know but never knew that I needed to know."

You will find that Mammoland is a place that is challenging and fascinating, remarkable and stressful, and can cause happiness and sadness all at the same time. I feel fortunate every day to be there. Participating in this process continues to be immensely satisfying for me personally and professionally. I have lived in Mammoland for many years and invite you in to see the remarkable world that it has become. Until there's a cure, there's Mammoland.

2

The Screening Mammogram Guidelines Controversy:

What You Absolutely Must Know

ADDRESSING THE ELEPHANT IN THE ROOM, AND

THE CASE FOR TOMOSYNTHESIS

THE RECENT CONTROVERSIAL recommendations by the U.S. Preventive Services Task Force (USPSTF) and the American Cancer Society (ACS) regarding screening mammograms have ignited a storm of outrage and scrutiny of the premise and science behind the benefits of screening mammography. The controversy has stimulated radiologists and other physicians and organizations involved in breast cancer care to clear the air, clarify the facts, and educate the public about this lifesaving test. According to Daniel Kopans at the 2016 meeting of the Society of Breast Imaging, the USPSTF and ACS recommendations are "very paternalistic" because they denote *anxiety* as a harm serious enough to recommend against or downgrade a lifesaving examination and portray the harm of anxiety derived from having the mammogram as greater than its lifesaving value.

American women are not weak, fragile beings who cannot take a bit of stress, especially to undergo an examination that could save their lives. In this chapter, I discuss the controversial recommendations and the science behind screening mammography, clarify the facts, and counter the arguments used to recommend against screening. I also give recommendations about how to proceed in the future.

Breast cancer is the most commonly diagnosed malignancy in women, and it is the second leading cause of cancer-related deaths among American women. As a result of improvements in treatment and early detection over the past 2 decades, millions of women are surviving breast cancer today. The current mortality rate for breast cancer is significantly lower than much higher rates that had previously remained unchanged for 50 years. Mammographic screening has been the crucial element in improving survival by allowing radiologists to identify cancers at earlier stages, which increases treatment success. Women with early-stage cancers confined to the breast have a 5-year survival rate of greater than 98%.

Unfortunately, in 2009 and 2016, the USPSTF withdrew its support for screening mammography for women between the ages of 40 and 49 and for women older than 75 years of age; and recommended that women 50 to 74 years of age be screened every 2 years instead of annually. They also recommended against **clinical breast examination** and **breast self-examination** (highlighted terms are defined in the Glossary). These changes are still producing negative effects and causing confusion among patients and health care providers.

Those of us who are involved in the early detection and treatment of breast cancer disagree with the USPSTF guidelines. The American College of Radiology (ACR), the Society of Breast Imaging (SBI), and the American College of Obstetrics and Gynecology (ACOG) strongly disagree with the recommendations. These institutions continue to recommend yearly screening mammography commencing at age 40 for the general population. Under these well-documented screening guidelines, we have seen a 35% drop in breast cancer deaths among women of all ages.

There are many problems with the USPSTF recommendations:

- The 16-member USPSTF had not one physician specializing in breast cancer screening, diagnosis, or treatment on its panel.
- Screening mammography is the most carefully scrutinized test in medical history, with 9 of the 10 worldwide, randomized, controlled screening trials showing a 30% to 44% overall decrease in breast cancer deaths among women offered screening mammography compared with women not offered screening; nonrandomized screening studies showed a decrease of up 63%.
- The benefit of the randomized trials would have been even greater if all of the women offered screening mammography in the study groups had undergone the examination. Up to 50% of women in this arm of the trials never accepted the invitation to be screened. All women in the screening group had to be counted in that group whether they underwent mammography or not; therefore, cancers developing in women who did not undergo the screening were counted together with those developing in women whose cancers were found on the screening mammograms. Because the cancers found in the women who were not screened were much larger when discovered, these women did not do as well, and many died of their disease. USPSTF disregarded these data, and reported only a 15% reduction in breast cancer deaths among women 40 to 49 years of age. The actual decrease in this age group was 23% to 44%.

- As reported in a 2012 news release, researchers at the Mayo Clinic found that the controversial USPSTF guidelines resulted in an almost 6% decline in mammography rates for women between 40 and 49 years of age, resulting in an estimated 54,000 fewer mammograms performed. This is regrettable because screening mammography has led to a 29% decrease in death rates in this age group, and if screening rates decline, more young women will die of this disease unnecessarily.
- The USPSTF claimed that **false-positive** examinations cause harm to patients by increasing pain and anxiety, but most screening mammograms relieve anxiety about breast cancer. For at least 90% of women undergoing screening mammography, examination results are good news.

There is no perfect test in medicine, and mammography is no exception. However, it is by far the best weapon we have in the fight against breast cancer, and it is a proven method. All organizations, even the USPSTF and ACS, understand that annual screening mammography starting at 40 years of age saves the most lives.

What the Research Shows

It is important to have a general understanding of the research so as to better evaluate the data that are presented in the media. Because the controversy about mammography has widespread and significant implications for the lives of many women, it should not be decided by whose argument appears to be most persuasive on a television show or in a magazine article. Advertising and political tactics further confuse the issue and may reflect a divide and silence the opposition strategy. The information about mammography is important enough to understand in some detail.

It is beneficial in this context to know how good research is done. Well-designed studies that result in reliable results are called randomized, controlled trials (RCTs). The design of such a study compares a group of women who are offered screening mammograms with a group of similar women who are not offered screening mammography. The two groups should be almost identical in every other way, including age and other demographics, medical history, and family history. These studies randomly assign patients to the two comparison groups (i.e., researchers do not designate subjects for a particular group). The groups are studied over the same period of time and under the same conditions. Over time, some of the women develop breast cancer. The researchers then determine the actual number of women in each group who were diagnosed with the disease. They record other data about each woman, such as her age at diagnosis, cancer stage at diagnosis (i.e., whether the disease has spread), what treatments she received as a result of her diagnosis (e.g., surgery, radiation, chemotherapy), and her survival status after the diagnosis (i.e., whether she died of breast cancer).

Six RCTs were performed from 1963 to 1988:

1. HIP New York, 1963–1969 (40–64 years of age)
2. Malmö, Sweden, 1976–1986 (45–69 years of age)
3. Swedish Two County Trial, 1979–1988 (40–74 years of age)
4. Edinburgh, Scotland, 1981–1985 (45–64 years of age)
5. Gothenburg, Sweden, 1982–1988 (40–59 years of age)
6. Canadian trial, 1980–2005 (40–59 years of age)

The first five studies showed a statistically significant (20% to 32%) reduction in mortality for women of all ages. A 1996 subanalysis of five Swedish studies showed a 29% reduction in mortality for patients 40 to 49 years of age.

The Canadian trial was the only one of these studies that did not show a reduction in mortality with the use of screening mammography. This finding reflects the protocols and research methods; the study was not randomized properly, although it was called an RCT. It was the only study that was not population based but instead relied on volunteers. It also placed an excessive number of symptomatic women in the screening group; by definition, these women should not have been included in the study at all. Because all women were given a physical examination before they were randomized, the investigators knew who was symptomatic and preferentially placed them in the group receiving mammograms! This went against all the tenants of a blinded review and stacked the deck for one group over another. The comparison groups were by definition not equal, and comparisons of unequal groups has no value.

Outside expert reviewers at the time of the Canadian study judged many of the mammograms as technically inadequate even by 1980 standards due to improper positioning, poor compression, faulty processing, and lack of mammographic grids. The technologists who performed the examinations were not trained in a standard technique to ensure quality or comparability of images from one study site to another. The radiologists who interpreted the films were not trained in the evaluation of mammograms or in a consistent method for documenting their findings. As a result, findings that were identical between patients might be described and reported differently by different radiologists. Therefore, the two similar findings would be calculated as different outcomes in the study. On the other hand, two totally different findings could be classified as similar.

The only thing the Canadian study proved was that poor mammography and poor protocol do not improve outcomes and are worse than having no mammography at all. Most breast cancer experts throw out this study when analyzing the effectiveness of screening mammography, but the USPSTF considered it as the premier study on which their recommendations were based! As the old adage says, garbage in equals garbage out, and evaluating the bad data 30 years later does not correct it.

Breast cancer–specific mortality rates (i.e., death rates attributed to breast cancer) were compared in a 29-year study of one half of the population of Sweden and reported by Tabar and colleagues in 2001. This review revealed a 63% reduction in the mortality rate for those between 40 and 69 years of age who underwent screening mammography when compared with women of similar age during the period before screening was available. In contrast, there was no change in the mortality rate for women 40 to 69 years of age who were not screened compared with women during that earlier time period. These findings strongly suggest that the lifesaving benefits resulted from screening and not from improved treatment.

In RCTs as a whole, the following numbers of women needed to be screened to save one woman's life by detecting early breast cancer:

Age 40–49: need to screen 746 women
Age 50–59: need to screen 351 women
Age 60–69: need to screen 233 women

As reported by Feig and coworkers in 2012, these numbers meet even the USPSTF standards to justify screening for all of the age categories.

Overdiagnosis Versus Overtreatment

In addition to the apparently crippling anxiety women may have from undergoing a screening mammogram, the USPSTF reported that another significant harm to women from getting screening mammograms is the possibility of overdiagnosis. This position ignores the rationale of identifying a cancer early so that it can be taken care of. The USPSTF argument about overdiagnosis stems from the possibility that some cancers are found at such an early stage (i.e., confined to the breast) and grade (i.e., few or no aggressive features) that in theory they may not ever progress to threaten the woman (i.e., breast cancer will not be the reason she dies). The cancer is so slow growing and has so many favorable characteristics that it will never become invasive, get into the bloodstream, metastasize to other organs, and cause death.

Proponents of this argument routinely quote low-grade **ductal carcinoma in situ (DCIS)** as the poster child for the theory of overdiagnosis. The literature does support a long-term survival rate of greater than 95% with mastectomy or lumpectomy plus radiation therapy and no chemotherapy. This suggests these cancers can be treated with less aggressive interventions and less debilitating treatments, reducing the side effects and complications and making the treatments less costly and less harmful to the patient. The cancer is treated or cured with the fewest complications by therapeutically conservative means because the situation does not require more elaborate treatment. There are specific protocols in the surgical and oncology specialties whereby women with early-stage breast cancer can be treated in a very conservative but effective manner with excellent results. Thus, it is evident that they are not *over*treated.

The treatment recommendations for these women, as for all breast cancer patients, should be individualized, with "less being more" if the outcomes are the same. This approach has played out over time for the transition of standard surgical management of breast cancer from radical mastectomy to lumpectomy plus radiation therapy: In most cases, the prognosis (i.e., how the patient fares in the long term) is the same.

However, the situation just described is not the same as overdiagnosis. Purposely not diagnosing a cancer that is detectable on the mammogram or not performing mammograms so that patients remain ignorant about the cancer (i.e., there is no test evidence because no image was obtained) is what proponents of overdiagnosis are asking us to do.

Some cancers are found at such an early stage that they are confined to the breast duct (Fig. 2.1). I use the analogy of cancer within a straw. The breast duct, which is the straw, has no holes. The cancer has no way to get outside of the straw and invade the surrounding breast tissue or gain access to blood or lymphatic vessels that would allow it to travel (i.e., metastasize) to other parts of the body. The risk of death from breast cancer correlates with its ability to metastasize. If breast cancers always remained confined to the breast, there would be no mortality associated with it.

We want to find the cancers as early as possible so as to save the most lives. This is the whole premise of screening with mammography when a woman is not having any symptoms. Fifty years ago, in comparison, cancers were discovered mainly by detection of a hard mass in the breast and were likely to have already metastasized to other parts of the body.

The current understanding is that in situ cancers, given enough time, can eventually progress to invasive cancers and make a hole in the straw, gaining access to the surrounding

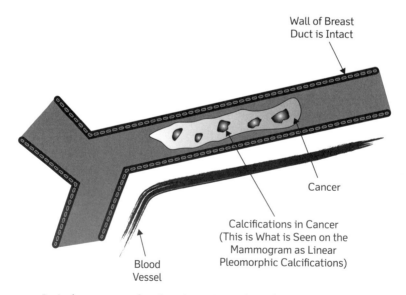

Wall of Breast
Duct is Intact

Cancer

Calcifications in Cancer
(This is What is Seen on the
Mammogram as Linear
Pleomorphic Calcifications)

Blood
Vessel

FIGURE 2.1 In situ breast cancer: ductal carcinoma in situ (DCIS).

tissue, where blood and lymphatic vessels can transport cancer cells to other parts of the body (Fig. 2.2). The timeframe that this requires (i.e., slow-growing vs. fast-growing), the level of invasion (i.e., to what extent the cancer has spread to surrounding tissues), and the propensity of the cancer to metastasize (i.e., travel in the bloodstream to other organs such as liver, bones, and brain) depend on the type of cancer and its activity pattern.

Breast cancer is a group of more than 20 types of tumors with different characteristics, behaviors, and outcomes. Some are very indolent and take years to grow to any substantial degree, whereas some are exceedingly aggressive and cause obvious changes in weeks to months. With the many advances in medical oncology, including genetic evaluation of cancer cells, much can be predicted about the behavior of a particular type of cancer. However, what has not been determined is which DCIS cancers in a given woman will or will not progress to invasive cancers. Telling you not to treat the disease is like telling you to just take your chances. Statistically, the likelihood of a DCIS becoming markedly aggressive in a short period is low, but why wait for it to become invasive when it could be treated and cured now?

At an early stage, treatment can be minimally invasive with few side effects, and the result is cure. It is foolish not treat a curable condition based on the argument that it should progress to a more lethal stage before being addressed. Moreover, there is no way to know which of these cancers will progress and which will not. Statistics do not tell us what will happen in an individual case. Although the medical fields of oncology and genetics are working diligently to provide better means of identification, that time is not here yet. It is unethical, if not immoral, to counsel someone to decline treatment of a

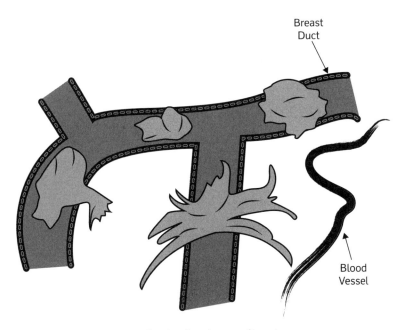

FIGURE 2.2 Invasive breast cancer, showing four degrees of invasion.

curable disease until the disease progresses to a point at which it threatens their life. We should be less concerned about overdiagnosis than overtreatment.

The Case for Tomosynthesis

Tomosynthesis (i.e., three-dimensional mammography) optimizes digital mammography by producing multiple slices or images through the breast tissue, allowing radiologists to see inside the breast tissue better. This technology was invented at Harvard and is one of the most important medical advances in the past 25 years. I think it will greatly improve our ability to detect early breast cancers.

Tomosynthesis can dramatically decrease the limitations and increase the benefits of screening mammography. Studies from Norway, Italy, and the United States show significant reductions in the number of false-positive mammograms (i.e., identifying lesions that turn out not to be cancer) and simultaneous increases in cancer detection rates (i.e., finding real cancers).

Work by Rose and colleagues has shown that the benefits of tomosynthesis are obtainable beyond the academic research setting and that they have widespread practical application. The benefit seen in their studies translates into real results in community practice, which is the realm in which most breast imaging is performed. The results showed a statistically significant reduction in recalls: 37% of women who would previously have been called back because of an abnormal mammogram did not get called back because the radiologist had enough information from the tomosynthesis to determine that the lesion was not cancer. On the other hand, the total cancer detection rate increased by 35%, and the detection of invasive cancers (i.e., those with the potential to metastasize) increased by 54%. Therefore, tomosynthesis is finding more cancers and, more significantly, it is finding more potentially deadly cancers at an earlier stage than with standard two-dimensional mammography.

Tomosynthesis addresses and corrects both of the harms the USPSTF cites as reasons for not supporting screening mammography: There are 37% fewer callbacks, and thus 37% fewer "anxious" women, and more cancers are actually diagnosed. The greatest benefit is detection of small but significant invasive cancers; this outweighs in importance the "overdiagnosis" of low-grade in situ cancers.

Misunderstanding the Recommendation of Risk-Based Screening with Mammography

The USPSTF and others argue that screening mammography should be risk based, meaning that the screening protocol should be individualized based on factors such as family history, age at menarche, and age at menopause. However, this approach to screening mammography for the general population is wrong. The two biggest risk factors for developing breast cancer are being a woman (i.e., gender) and getting older (i.e., age). More than 75% of women who are diagnosed with breast cancer have no additional risk factors other than being a woman and getting older. If the USPSTF's flawed reasoning were followed, we would screen only the 25% of women who have additional risk factors. This means that, like 50 years ago, the other 75% would be kept waiting until their cancers were more advanced before they became aware of the disease. The USPSTF approach would erase all of the advancements in medical science related to early detection of breast cancer and improved survival.

Appropriate risk-based screening means adding supplemental examinations to the mammogram screening protocol, including discussion of breast density and risk assessment for high-risk patients. However, this is not appropriate for average-risk women (i.e., all women older than 40 years of age). There are no known factors that can downgrade a woman's risk and remove her from the list of those who should be screened. Screening mammography should be performed annually for all women starting at age 40 years or sooner if the woman has risk factors that require earlier or more in-depth screening. In no circumstance does a woman's risk profile justify starting at an older age or having less frequent screening.

RADIOLOGY CONSULT

The facts are straightforward. Screening mammography has been proven to be a lifesaving test. Annual screening starting at 40 years of age saves the most lives. Variations and recommendations to the contrary will result in more deaths from breast cancer. Women can go along with the USPSTF's paternalistic opinion that the harms of anxiety and theoretical overdiagnosis are legitimate reasons not have a potentially lifesaving test, but I think women are smarter and certainly strong-willed enough to get a screening mammogram every year beginning at age 40.

II

The Who

3

You! How You Impact Your Care

YOUR RESPONSIBILITIES AND INFORMATION

YOU NEED TO KNOW

BEING A PATIENT is not a passive endeavor, and nowhere is this more evident than in breast imaging. How you interact with staff, what you know about your situation, what you bring to the appointment, and what actions you take all affect the outcome of the evaluation. Patients have responsibilities to provide medical, procedural, and family histories, such as details of previous biopsies or operations. You should bring prior films and reports with you and be prepared to describe symptom characteristics concisely and accurately. What is the finding? When did it start? Is it stable or changing? How long has it been there? The best and most accurate outcomes depend on the full and active participation by the patient, who should be as interested in their care as the providers are.

This chapter emphasizes the importance of patient responsibilities, such as retrieving prior films, knowing your medical and family histories, paying attention during the referring physician visit, knowing your current health status, taking responsibility for follow-up, making realistic scheduling plans, and having a cooperative attitude.

Retrieval of Prior Films

You should be prepared to retrieve old films and reports. This is an essential step in the evaluation process, and it can be a determining factor in deciding whether a biopsy is needed. Lack of this step adds a considerable amount of additional work for the facility. The radiologist may have to re-read the study (not an efficient use of time or resources) if the films come in weeks after the evaluation. If they are never retrieved the radiologist may be forced to base her decision on the available information alone, possibly leading to an unnecessary biopsy.

It is in your best interest to make the effort. I have had patients refuse to retrieve old films just because they did not feel like it. Really. Do not assume that gathering your prior data is someone else's responsibility. The health care provider has no way of knowing the name of the facility described as the "one with the blue roof near the grocery store." It is unacceptable to ask for an evaluation and then handicap the health care personnel by not providing data that could assist in the evaluation.

Absence of prior films could affect your workup in several ways:

It may obligate the radiologist to read your films as a first-time (i.e., baseline) examination; as a result, you do not get the benefit that review of the old films would provide.

It may require you to have an additional workup with mammography, ultrasound, or **magnetic resonance imaging (MRI)** for a finding that has already been studied or is stable (highlighted terms are defined in the Glossary).

It may require you to have a biopsy of a lesion that has been biopsied before.

It may lead to delay or rescheduling of a biopsy because not enough information is known about what another facility reported to do the procedure at the current facility.

It may be based on the erroneous assumption that all digital mammograms can be accessed by any facility because they are computer based and must be linked; in actuality, the radiologist has no access to private information at another facility.

It may result from not understanding that targeting for biopsy usually requires review of the previous image itself, not just the report. In some cases, to proceed with the scheduled biopsy, the current facility must repeat the entire study, which adds additional cost and time.

These situations are most stressful when there is a time limit, such as when the patient is scheduled for surgery in 2 days and the information is needed to plan the correct type of surgery or when the patient is planning to go out of the country for 4 months. Rescheduling of a follow-up examination may be required if the initial films were done elsewhere and not at the current facility. Knowing what finding to pursue requires review of the previous outside films; in some cases, the entire study may need to be repeated if the physician is forced for some reason to proceed with the follow-up evaluation on that day.

If there are known prior studies, I am comfortable waiting 2 to 3 weeks for them to arrive for comparison purposes. If they do not become available, I dictate an addendum report and base my recommendation on the available information and the current study alone. By this time, the assumption is that the prior information is not available or cannot be retrieved, and I must proceed in a timely fashion with the findings of the current study.

Tips for film retrieval include the following:

Start early. If it is close to the time for your screening examination, try to start 1 month in advance in your search. This will increase the likelihood that the films will arrive in time to take them to your examination.

If you have questions or need advice, call the radiology file room at the facility that you will be going to, and they may be able to assist you. They may have a database of facility names, especially if the previous films were taken at another facility in your area.

If you do not recall the name of the previous facility, inquire at the office of your previous doctor; the staff members usually can access the report, which will have the name of the facility.

It is best to pick the films up yourself, or you can have them mailed to you or to the new breast imaging facility.

If the examination was a film screen, ask for original films, not copies. Compact discs containing this information can easily be uploaded into the computer system at the new facility.

Ask for printed reports in addition. The history or recommendations documented on the report may be relevant to the current examination and may determine the type of study that is performed

Bring all of your breast imaging films and reports with you on the day of your examination.

Know Your Family History

Although most breast imaging centers do not perform formal genetic risk assessments, information that you provide about your family history can affect the workup. (For example, both breast cancer and ovarian cancer are associated with mutated *BRCA1* and *BRCA2* genes.) It is important to know your family history in regard to first-degree relatives (e.g., mother, sister, daughter) and second-degree relatives (e.g., cousin, aunt, grandmother). Information about your paternal (father's) side is just as important as that about your maternal (mother's) side. For example, your father might carry a mutated gene, which could have been passed on to you, but might not develop the disease himself because the effect is much less in men than in women. The age of your relatives at the time of their cancer diagnosis and whether they were premenopausal (i.e., before menopause) or postmenopausal (i.e., having "gone through the change") is also relevant.

Your family history is considered in the context of an imaging workup:

You may be deemed to be an appropriate candidate for additional imaging studies, such as screening ultrasound or screening MRI.

Your history may warrant a mammographic evaluation even if you would not get one based on the usual age criteria.

You may need to commence annual screening mammograms before 40 years of age.

In the case of borderline findings, the family history may tilt the balance toward biopsy rather than simple follow-up.

The data may prompt consultation with a genetics counseling service for possible testing.

Know Your Breast Health History

At some point in their lives, many women have breast procedures and biopsies. Some procedures cause no alteration of the breast tissue that is perceptible on imaging studies, but others produce findings that are evident on imaging studies. Knowing which type of procedure or biopsy you had helps the radiologist correlate the findings on the film with the history. The technologist usually asks for this information before the examination and marks any identifiable skin scars, alerting the radiologist to the history during evaluation of the films.

The radiologist compares the imaging findings with the stated history—if they correlate, great. If the separate facts do not correspond, additional investigation will be necessary to further characterize the finding. For example, a patient states that she has had a **surgical biopsy** in the right *upper* outer aspect of the breast, and a scar marker placed in that region is visible on the mammogram film, but the film shows a distortion in the right *lower* outer aspect the breast. The surgical history does not explain the presence of distortion in this other area, so the finding is suspicious and warrants further evaluation to exclude a cancer. On the other hand, if the distortion is in the right upper aspect of the breast, the surgical history explains the imaging finding, and no further workup is needed because it is an *expected* finding.

Some breast-related histories can cause an altered appearance on imaging:

Needle biopsy: Usually, there is no visible scar, but scars have become more frequently encountered with vacuum-assisted techniques because of the increased amount of tissue retrieved (which is a good thing).

Excisional biopsy: A scar is usually seen, but it can be subtle.

Lumpectomy: The scar and surgical bed are usually evident as an obvious distortion and density; surgical clips frequently are seen in the lumpectomy site.

Prior radiation therapy: Irradiation usually causes thickening of the trabeculae (i.e., strands) within the breast tissue and usually causes skin thickening.

Mastectomy: There may be some residual fatty tissue that can be imaged if requested by the referring physician or if this has been the patient's routine.

Implant placement, revision, or explantation (implant removal): The radiologist may see the implant capsule (i.e., fibrous scar), a distortion, or free silicone.

Reduction or **lift**: There is a typical distortion pattern after these procedures.

Knowing the general time frame of previous procedures helps the radiologist to know whether acute healing changes related to the area should be seen (which otherwise could simulate disease). Knowing that a surgical procedure was recently performed assists in understanding what the expected finding should be, thus decreasing the potential for "overcall."

Seeing Your Referring Doctor

Although it is the referring doctor's responsibility to provide a sufficient history when ordering an examination, physicians frequently place an order for a breast evaluation with only a vague history such as "breast lump"—no commentary about location, size, or distance from the nipple. Calling the office for clarification during a busy workday is usually futile, and it is almost impossible to get someone in the referring doctor's office to stop other tasks, pull the chart, review the chart, and then call back with the details (if there has been anything written in the chart at all) while the patient is still at the facility—especially if it is an hour past time for her study and she needs to pick up her kids from school in 30 minutes. I counsel you to pay attention.

When your physician is concerned enough to send you for a study based on a finding on the **clinical breast examination (CBE)**, notice where the breast was palpated. Ask to be shown where the questionable area is located, and have the doctor explain why it warrants evaluation. Then, when you come in for the diagnostic imaging evaluation, you can point out the area of concern and the assessment can be more precisely targeted to that area. Occasionally, referring physicians mark the area of concern with a marker (i.e., X on the skin) and ask the patient to leave it there until the visit to the breast center. Either way, you, as a patient, should be interested to know this information and not passively accept *breast lump* as a diagnosis. The outcome, good or bad, most significantly affects you.

Information to Know About Your Current Status

Giving a concise and relevant history about your symptoms helps your doctor, the technologist, and the radiologist to better assess your condition, and from a radiology standpoint, it determines the type of examination to be performed.

Information to report about your current status includes the following:

Do you have a symptom or problem, or are you asymptomatic (i.e., without symptoms)?

If you have a problem or symptom, is it acute (i.e., new) or chronic (i.e., long-standing)? When did it start?

Has this symptom been addressed with your doctor? Has it been previously evaluated with imaging? Has it been previously biopsied?

Does it change or fluctuate (i.e., come and go)? Is it associated with your menstrual cycle?

Is it increasing, decreasing, or staying the same?

Do you have any associated findings?

Have you had trauma to the area?

Be Responsible for Completing the Recommended Plan of Action:

After an evaluation is complete, the radiologist states the conclusion of the findings and renders an opinion as to the disposition (plan of action) based on established standards of care, history, experience, and so on. You now have the option to agree or disagree with the recommendation.

If you agree with a recommendation, follow it. If you do not agree, just say no. Informed refusal is the acceptable and preferred way to decline a procedure or recommendation (Box 3.1). There are sometimes legitimate and logical reasons to decline a recommended course of action, or you may just not want to do it. Either way, ignoring correspondence (which wastes resources and staff time) or repeatedly scheduling and then not showing up for the appointment is not an acceptable way to handle this interaction. If you are unsure or unclear, ask for further clarification. Be inquisitive. Ask a lot of questions: "Doctor, why do you recommend that course of action? What are the alternatives? What will happen if I do nothing? What is the worse-case scenario?"

Scheduling and Other Housekeeping Issues

Have your order with you, or confirm that it has been received in advance of your visit. Radiologists are consult physicians; orders for examinations must come from another physician except in specific circumstances, such as screening programs that allow self-referrals. Most facilities will not start the examination until an order is confirmed.

If you are already scheduled for implant surgery or are going out of town, plan accordingly when scheduling your screening examination. Schedule far enough in advance to allow time to come back for additional views (i.e., diagnostic study) or a biopsy if necessary. Scheduling the evaluation for the day before you are to have surgery is not wise. Failure to schedule properly may result in delay of your surgery or travel plans—or, even worse, proceeding with implant surgery without a full evaluation of the area in question, which could be cancer.

BOX 3.1
REFUSAL TO CONSENT FOR DIAGNOSTIC PROCEDURE/IMAGING FORM

1. I hereby refuse and decline, voluntarily and freely, to consent to the following procedure/imaging:

_____

2. I am (or the patient is) unable (i.e., due to incapacity or minor status) or unwilling to consent to this procedure/imaging for the following reasons:

_____

3. I understand that this procedure/imaging is recommended by the ordering physician and/or the attending radiologist based on the assessment of my health history and/or my imaging results.

4. I understand that there are potential serious negative consequences of my refusal to undergo this procedure/imaging. The consequences include, but are not limited to, improper diagnosis of my condition, failure to detect or diagnose a new serious condition in a timely fashion, and loss of a chance to successfully treat and/or cure a serious condition due to delay in diagnosis.

5. After being informed of the above risks of not proceeding with this procedure/imaging, I hereby fully and permanently release this facility and its affiliates and employees, the attending radiologist, and all others participating in my care from any and all present and future legal claims related to my refusal of the proposed procedure/imaging.

6. I understand that I may later change my mind and return to the ordering physician for another order for the procedure/imaging. This facility will make best efforts to reschedule this procedure/imaging.

My signature below attests my refusal to consent to this procedure/imaging.

_____

(Signature of Patient/Representative)

_____

Modified from MICA Insurance Company, Phoenix, Arizona.

View your visit as a doctor's appointment, not a run to the carwash for service. Although your examination is scheduled for a specific time and the provider makes every effort to stay caught up, it is rare to have no delays; schedules effectively hold your place in line. In the practice of medicine, there are numerous factors that alter even the best plans (e.g., late patients, which delay all subsequent examinations; debilitated or frail patients who take longer to accommodate; waiting for orders to be faxed; tearful patients who need consoling; urgent add-on cases; emergencies; surgical patients). If you are the patient who needs extra time to discuss your findings, we will take the time with you as well. So, be reasonable and compassionate with others, understanding and patient. When seen you will receive the individualized care that you need too.

Allot enough time in your schedule to have the examination performed. Routine screening mammograms take about 15 minutes (for performance of the examination only). Paperwork, changing clothes, history taking, and other factors should also be accounted for during planning. Diagnostic examinations may take 30 minutes to 2 hours to perform, depending on the complexity of the findings and what additional studies are needed. Call to inquire about the time that will be required for the examination if you are unsure. Do not schedule your appointment for a diagnostic evaluation at 1 PM and your appointment to get your hair colored at 1:30 PM.!

Personality Issues

Having a bad day? We all have them, but taking it out on the radiology staff is detrimental to the evaluation process. Rushing the technologist, pulling back, and being tense negatively impact the technical outcome of the study (i.e., the quality of your films), which in turn impacts the ability of the radiologist to detect abnormalities. Appreciate that the evaluation is being performed to benefit you and that assisting in the process helps you to get the best examination possible. Your cooperation in the process is needed to optimize the evaluation.

If you have any problems, you should contact the mammography supervisor or breast health navigator.

You! A Quick List

- Get old films in advance.
- Know your family history.
- Know your breast health history, including biopsies.
- Be informed about your visit to your referring doctor.
- Know your current health status, including symptoms.
- Bring an order for your examination.
- Schedule enough time to have your evaluation completed.
- Bring a cooperative attitude.
- Ask questions if you have concerns.

RADIOLOGY CONSULT

The old adage, "You only get out of something what you put into it," holds true in breast imaging. Inaccurate or absent information can lead to an incorrect or incomplete assessment. This is not a situation in which a reported laboratory value can provide the answer. History taking and information gathering require the active participation of several people (including you) at several junctures. What you bring to the table and the accuracy of that information influence the workup. Be an active participant in your health. It really does matter.

4

The Breast Imaging Team

RADIOLOGIST, TECHNOLOGIST, AND NAVIGATOR

THE BREAST IMAGING team is led by the **radiologist** (i.e., physician imaging expert) and includes the navigator, **radiologic technologist**, technologist supervisor, and many other critical support personnel, including administrative, clerical, and clinical staff and the medical physicist (highlighted terms are defined in the Glossary). The coordinated efforts of all of these participants enable delivery of high-quality medical care and efficient service for the patient. This chapter describes the training and education requirements and basic functions of a few of these staff members, most notably the radiology physician, who has a minimum of 13 years of postgraduate education in the field of medical imaging.

The Radiologist

A radiologist is a specialist medical doctor who is trained in medical image interpretation and the performance of radiologic procedures to diagnose and treat diseases—just as a cardiologist is a physician trained in the assessment of heart conditions and the performance of cardiac procedures. The radiologist's education begins with a 4-year college degree (i.e., BA or BS), after which he or she takes an entrance examination, the Medical College Admission Test (MCAT), and applies to medical school. Medical school is traditionally a 4-year experience that educates the student in the basics of modern medicine, including anatomy, physiology, pharmacology, pathophysiology, and pathology. On satisfactory completion, the student graduates with a Doctor of Medicine (M.D.) or Doctor of Osteopathic Medicine (D.O.) degree.

The new doctor then chooses a medical specialty (e.g., obstetrics and gynecology, pediatrics, surgery, radiology) and applies to residency training programs that are designed to teach the details of that area of medicine. The candidate chooses multiple programs, and the programs select multiple candidates based on the their applications, references, grades, and other factors. A computer analyzes this information and finds the best matches based on the candidates' and the program's ranking preferences. After much anticipation, the results are announced on Match Day.

During this time, the student must also take and pass a standard licensing test, the U.S. Medical Licensing Examination (USMLE). The new doctor who aspires to be a radiologist must complete a 1-year clinical internship to gain a basic practical knowledge about general medicine, surgery, or a combination of both. The doctor then enters a radiology residency program. The radiology residency is a 4-year training period during which the doctor is educated about all aspects of medical imaging in many areas of medicine. During this period, the resident performs and interprets tens of thousands of examinations and receives extensive didactic training from faculty. At the end of the training, the doctor is awarded a certificate of satisfactory completion of residency and has the necessary hours of instruction required to practice in the field of diagnostic radiology.

The doctor is then considered board eligible and has the requirements needed to sit for a series of examinations that must be passed to become board certified by the American Board of Radiology. This certification acknowledges that the practicing radiologist has satisfied the requirements of the Board, meets the minimum standards of the organization, and is deemed to be competent in the field of medical imaging. Unlike some other specialties in medicine, employers almost always require radiologists to be board certified, not just board eligible.

At this point, the radiologist can interview for jobs and work independently as a practicing radiology specialist. Many radiologists voluntarily complete additional fellowship training to become subspecialized in a particular area of medical imaging (e.g., interventional, neuroradiology, pediatrics, nuclear medicine). For example, I completed an additional year of intensive training in clinical breast imaging and mammography. Radiologists who interpret mammograms must continue to read a designated number of films to stay eligible to do this work. They also must participate in ongoing continuing medical education (CME) programs to maintain the ability to read mammograms and other medical imaging studies and to meet maintain licensure requirements to practice medicine in the state.

Although radiology in general allows for ample intellectual stimulation and constant technologic innovations in the field (keeping the work exciting and very satisfying), breast imaging adds the advantage of patient interaction that further increases personal and professional satisfaction. Interaction with patients and doctors increases the accuracy of the assessment of the radiologic examinations and also adds a multidisciplinary component to the approach to care by involving doctors of different specialties in management and treatment planning. For these reasons, I think breast imaging is one of the most satisfying areas of medicine. It is wonderful to find a career that matches and enhances your strengths and personality. Lucky me!

The Navigator

The **breast patient navigator** includes a broad spectrum of medical specialists including nurses, technologists, social workers, primary care providers, etc. These highly trained professionals can be certified as breast patient navigators for imaging and cancer (CN-BN). This is a relatively new subspecialization. Navigators are certified as breast patient navigators by organizations such as the National Consortium of Breast Centers (NCBC), an organization that started its certification program in 2008. Rigorous testing and credentialing is required to obtain this distinct designation.

The progress made in breast imaging and treatment of breast disease has been substantial, and the process often seems quite complex and overwhelming to patients. Working in communication with the radiologists, the patient's health care providers, and the resources within the community, navigators are available to facilitate procedures, educate patients regarding their imaging, clarify a diagnosis and the possible treatment plan, and support and refer patients to medical, community, and social support resources that eliminate barriers and meet their needs. To maintain certification, the navigator must obtain continuing education units (CEUs) specific to breast imaging, breast cancer, and professional skills related to breast care patients.

The concept of navigation was started by Dr. Harold P. Freeman in Harlem in 1990. Navigation can begin even prior to the diagnosis of breast cancer and continues throughout the continuum of care into survivorship.

The Radiologic Technologist

In breast imaging, the radiologic technologists (RTs) are medical personnel who perform the examinations (i.e., mammograms, ultrasound scans, and magnetic resonance imaging). According to their governing organization, the American Society of Radiologic Technologists (ASRT), RTs are "educated in anatomy, patient positioning, examination techniques, equipment protocols, radiation safety, radiation protection, and basic patient care." Certified RTs must complete at least 2 years of formal training at an accredited hospital-based program or a 2- or 4-year program at an academic institution. They also must pass a national certification examination and maintain ongoing licensure and continuing education credits to continue to perform examinations.

Mammographers are RTs who have additional training and whose primary focus is performing mammograms. They use x-rays to produce a mammographic image. They must meet strict educational and hands-on clinical training criteria as mandated by the Mammography Quality Standards Act (MQSA) of 1992.

The skills of RTs in properly positioning the patient for the mammogram and their knowledge of imaging techniques allow them to provide quality images to the radiologist for interpretation. High-quality films are essential for the most accurate interpretation.

If the imaging is suboptimal, the interpretation may be limited. For example, if there is motion on the film, calcifications could easily be missed because the film is blurry. If the posterior tissue (i.e., tissue close to the chest wall) is not on the image, a lesion in that area cannot be detected. The condition and cooperation of the patient and the skill of the technologist play critical roles in the ultimate quality of the image that reaches the radiologist.

Breast ultrasound technologists are RTs who have additional training and specialize in ultrasound of the breast. They produce images by placing an ultrasound transducer on the breast to look for abnormalities. The sound waves are converted into an image that is displayed on a monitor for evaluation by the technologist. **Ultrasound** (also called sonography) is very user dependent and requires the interpretive skills of the sonographer, who finds lesions and determines whether they are significant. They must also distinguish normal anatomy from abnormal findings.

In most facilities, the ultrasound technologist performs the examination and the radiologist interprets the static images. At some facilities, the radiologist directly evaluates the patient in real time. At my institution, the radiologists frequently perform the ultrasound examinations themselves or in addition to the ultrasound technologist.

RADIOLOGY CONSULT

The breast imaging team is a group of highly educated, well-qualified professionals with unique skills in the various aspects of the imaging process, from image acquisition to interpretation. This high degree of clinical expertise and the coordinated efforts of many other administrative and support personnel enable the breast imaging process to work effectively. A tremendous amount of effort and thought is invested in providing the highest degree of clinical care to patients.

5

The Rulers of Mammoland

MQSA, ACR, SBI, AND THE OTHER ABCS OF IMAGING

BREAST IMAGING IS one of the most regulated areas of medicine. Federal and state agencies oversee everything from film quality to physicians' recall rates and the number of cancers detected by a facility.

Mammography centers must be certified according to the **Mammography Quality Standards and Satisfaction Act of 1992 (MQSA)** and by the **American College of Radiology (ACR)**. The U.S. Food and Drug Administration (FDA) began inspections of mammography facilities to ensure MQSA compliance in January 1995.

MQSA, which became effective on October 1, 1994, was enacted by the U.S. Congress to regulate the quality of care in mammography, to meet uniform quality standards, and to maintain high-quality mammography in the United States and its territories. One of the most significant benefits of implementing MQSA was to legitimize direct communication between the radiologist and the patient. This federal mandate has helped to substantially decrease miscommunication or noncommunication of test results; it has significantly improved the radiologist's ability to deliver information, allowing the patient to receive unfiltered information directly from the radiologist. Women no longer have to have the information interpreted and distributed by their referring physician, and the data are delivered to the patient regardless of whether the referring physician believes it was relevant. This represents a momentous advance in patients' rights.

Breast imaging programs can voluntarily submit to a more rigorous standard and become Centers of Excellence (COE), a high distinction. The national practice standards for breast imaging are largely based on the ACR Appropriateness Criteria, which provides evidence-based guidelines for national practice standards to assist radiologists and other providers in making the most appropriate imaging or treatment decisions for a specific clinical condition.

To standardize reporting and provide clarity in the communication of test results and recommendations, the ACR developed the **Breast Imaging Reporting and Data System (BIRADS)**. This quality assurance tool provides guidelines for radiologists on how to describe findings and convey information about the test in understandable language.

The **Society of Breast Imaging (SBI)** is the only national organization dedicated exclusively to the support and advancement of breast imaging. Established in 1985, this organization of 3000 radiologists, medical physicists, and technologists exhibits a passionate dedication to saving lives through early detection of breast cancer.

RADIOLOGY CONSULT

Mammography is one of the most studied and most scrutinized specialties in recent medical history.

6

Your Referring Doctor

THE DELICATE BALANCE OF THE REFERRAL-CONSULT

RELATIONSHIP

RADIOLOGY IS A consulting specialty. This means that the radiologist is not the doctor who orders the examinations that he or she performs and interprets. Radiologists must in essence get permission from the referring physician to perform the examination. Although laws and programs allow asymptomatic women of appropriate age to self-refer and receive a screening mammogram without an order from a doctor, most breast examinations are ordered (i.e., prescribed) by another doctor or health care provider such as a physician's assistant or nurse practitioner. A provider refers the patient to a radiologist, as denoted by the term *referring physician* or *referring provider*.

Although health care providers order the examinations, their training is not in radiology. Most primary care physicians have extremely busy clinical practices with large patient loads and have limited time to thoroughly review the rapidly advancing and changing literature regarding current trends and recommendations in mammography and breast imaging. This problem has been confounded by controversies regarding American Cancer Society (ACS) and U.S. Preventive Services Task Force (USPSTF) mammography screening recommendations, which have led to confusion, uncertainty, and variation in ordering practices. The depth of knowledge referring doctors have about this subject largely depends on how interested they are in the topic, how aggressively they pursue continuing medical education on the subject, and what their relationship is with the local breast radiologist. This broad range of knowledge results in countless variations in practice and ordering styles. Some physicians order screening mammograms for patients with palpable breast lumps and assume that a negative mammographic result sufficiently excludes malignancy. Others submit orders for every asymptomatic patient to undergo a diagnostic examination because they want "to do everything for the patient" and/or to protect themselves from legal liability.

Although the ultimate goal of the referring physician is to provide the best care for a patient, misunderstandings about breast imaging can complicate the process. A referring physician may add unnecessary steps or otherwise hinder the process such that the standard of care to be performed as directed by the radiologist is limited. The time that the patient spends in the breast center can be significantly extended by trying to contact the referring physician or office staff to get corrected orders so that the radiologist can complete the evaluation on the scheduled day instead of having the patient return for another visit.

Patients may refuse certain examinations because the referring physician has counseled them incorrectly. This squanders the time of both the breast center's and the referring physician's staff, and it impedes the relationship of the patient and radiologist. The patient may think she has to choose between her referring physician and the radiologist. She has an established relationship with her referring doctor based on respect and trust and therefore may assume that her doctor would have ordered an ultrasound study if she truly needed one. Better overall communication between the radiologist and the referring physician produces more complete and accurate evaluations, and patients will have more confidence in the entire process.

The role of the referring physician is to assess the patient and provide an order with the history, symptoms, or physical examination findings that substantiate the type of examination being ordered. Does the patient need a screening evaluation or a diagnostic (problem-solving) study?

Some referring physicians tend to be either overreactors or underreactors. Radiologists commonly encounter discrepant orders such as an order for a screening mammogram when the patient has a breast lump. If this order were followed without question, the patient would not get the directed, specialized mammographic evaluation or ultrasound scan that is necessary in this clinical setting, and the likelihood of making an accurate diagnosis would be reduced. Referring physicians also commonly order a diagnostic examination for a patient with no symptoms because the doctor wants everything done for the patient. However, this can harm the patient because inconsequential lesions may be detected that must be investigated with a biopsy or followed, creating additional patient anxiety and increased health care expense. The responsible use of limited health care resources is a significant issue.

An important responsibility of the referring physician is to confirm that a patient undergoing screening is truly asymptomatic or has no acute or concerning problems and that her examination findings are negative. Radiologists assume that a screening patient has negative physical examination findings and a benign breast symptom history.

Referring physicians should have a method of follow-up to ensure that the ordered examinations are actually performed. They must also review the radiologist's report and act accordingly regarding the patient's care.

I prefer and advocate that referring physicians send orders for a breast imaging consultation similar to those they would write when consulting a cardiologist. They should include authorization for the radiologist to recall the patient from a screening examination, to perform a diagnostic mammogram and/or ultrasound study if warranted or based on the patient's symptoms, and to perform a needle-guided biopsy if it is needed for a tissue diagnosis. As the doctor who oversees the entire imaging process from screening to diagnosis, the radiologist is the only physician who is trained and skilled enough to determine which tests are needed to assess the patient, interpret the images, and make recommendations about the further course of action to be taken (i.e., disposition).

With breast radiologists becoming increasingly clinically oriented, the usefulness of the consult for the patient and the referring physician is greatly enhanced. This leads to superior patient care, greater patient satisfaction, and more accurate outcomes because it is a thorough and medically sound approach. No referring physician would send a patient to a cardiologist and then micromanage the entire process by deciding at every step what can or cannot be done for the patient. The same logic also applies to breast imaging and the radiology consultation. As with a cardiologist, if the referring physician's confidence in the specialist is that low, the patient should be sent elsewhere, to someone whose clinical assessment and management skills the doctor trusts. I think this is just as important in breast imaging. The clinical assessment and management skills of the radiologist and the quality of the facility make a difference for all diagnostic and screening patients.

RADIOLOGY CONSULT

Many of the issues for radiologists and referring physicians are matters of common sense. Some are more difficult to address than others because of egos, turf issues, and perceived control of the patient. Better communication and understanding of the process can alleviate many areas of controversy, but doctors do not always play well together.

III

The What

A picture is worth ten thousand words.

FRED R. BARNARD

7

The Tools of Breast Imaging

A PICTURE IS WORTH A THOUSAND WORDS

THIS CHAPTER REVIEWS the basic principles, merits, and limitations of the most commonly used breast imaging tests: mammography, ultrasound, and magnetic resonance imaging (MRI). The significance of image-guided biopsy as a tool used in patient care is explored briefly here but discussed in greater detail in Chapter 12. How each modality is used to address a clinical situation and when it should be employed in the workup are examined, but technical minutia are avoided.

Technically optimal images are the goal, but the technical performance of an examination may be limited for legitimate reasons. For instance, in mammography, the patient's condition (e.g., fragile, elderly), physical status (e.g., kyphotic, obese, restricted shoulder mobility), mental condition (e.g., impaired mental capacity due to a stroke, mental retardation), or emotional state (e.g., anxiety because a friend was recently diagnosed with breast cancer) can limit her ability to actively participate and may alter the optimal technical performance of the examination. For some patients, there is no way around these limitations, and after the radiologist's best efforts (with proper documentation of the limitations), the resulting films are considered to be the best that can be obtained. Still, they can have some interpretive value because they can provide some data. The study will be interpreted "as is" by the radiologist.

Methods of Breast Examination
MAMMOGRAPHY

In mammographic examinations, X-rays (i.e., low-dose radiation) are sent through the breast tissue, and an image is made of the breast. A very low dose of radiation is used, and compression of breast tissue during the examination is necessary for adequate visualization of findings. The resulting picture (i.e., **mammogram**) is a flat, two-dimensional representation of the breast tissue; on the mammogram, fatty areas are gray and dense areas are white (highlighted terms are defined in the Glossary). See Figure 7.1.

Mammography is the initial method of evaluation used because it detects the most abnormalities. This workhorse of breast imaging provides the point of reference from which most evaluations begin. It is the only test that has been proven to decrease **mortality** (death) from breast cancer.

Film-screen mammography: This traditional method of acquiring mammograms consists of a cassette (with a piece of film in it) that captures the image. The film is then run through a processor and developed in a manner similar to that used for darkroom photography.

Digital mammography: The images are acquired and displayed using computer-based technology that allows for manipulation of the images by the radiologist, which may result in better interpretations and fewer recalls. This method

CC

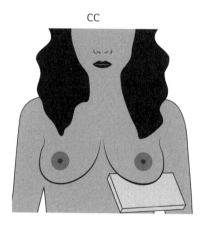

MLO

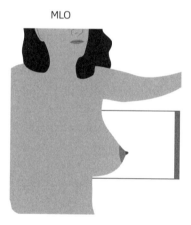

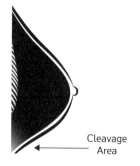

Cleavage
Area

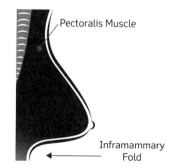

Pectoralis Muscle

Inframammary
Fold

FIGURE 7.1 Mammogram image.

was found in a large, multisite study to have an advantage over film-screen mammography for evaluating younger women and women with dense breasts. Digital mammography is the standard of care in most facilities.

Tomosynthesis (i.e., three-dimensional [3-D] mammography) consists of multiple, thin-slice mammographic images that allow the radiologist to see deep inside the breast. It is similar to computed tomography (CT) in that the radiologist can see inside the body at different depths. So, rather than two to three images per breast, tomosynthesis can provide 150 to 200 pictures per breast, which supplies a considerable amount of additional information. See Figure 7.2.

Tomosynthesis generates the "optimal" mammogram. Although it is useful for all breast densities, it is especially helpful for examination of women with dense breasts. Good research and the use of screening 3-D mammography in community settings have confirmed that tomosynthesis produces at least a 30% decrease in recalls (because areas of concern can be ruled out as suspicious with the available information). Abnormal lesions are seen better, and some are seen only on tomographic images, increasing the detection of small invasive cancers by 40%.

As the person who interprets the examination, I can tell you that 3-D mammography has improved my confidence level in reporting results as benign and my detection rate for finding subtle lesions. If I were queen, all eligible women of screening age would have a 3-D screening mammogram!

Contrast Mammography: With this procedure contrast dye is injected similar to MRI and digital mammographic images are acquired. Early research shows that this may be an

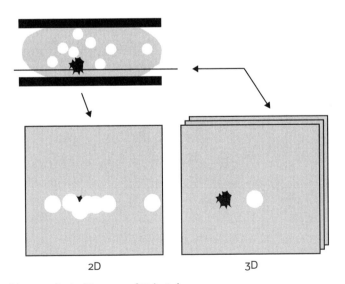

2D   3D

FIGURE 7.2 Tomosynthesis. (Courtesy of Hologic.)

alternative study for patients who are unable to undergo preoperative MRI (pacemaker, etc.) or further enhance the diagnostic usefulness of mammography.

ULTRASOUND

Ultrasound, also called *sonography*, uses sound waves to generate an image. A technologist or the radiologist puts a probe on the skin, which is used to see inside the breast tissue. Ultrasound is used primarily to determine whether a lesion is filled with fluid (i.e., **cyst**) or is solid (i.e., **tumor**). It commonly is used as an adjunct (i.e., helper) test to better characterize a mammographic finding or to detect palpable lesions even if the mammogram does not show an abnormality. Ultrasound is used increasingly as a supplemental screening examination (i.e., screening or survey ultrasound) in addition to screening mammography, especially for women with dense breast tissue. See Figure 7.3.

Ultrasound is user dependent, meaning that it is only as good as the person performing the examination because true lesions can be overlooked and other lesions can be falsely identified depending on the experience of the sonographer. Having an experienced and well-trained technologist who works with the radiologist is essential. Some companies offer automated ultrasound devices that lessen the user dependency of the examination, and these devices are beginning to be used in some academic and community settings. The jury is still out regarding its efficacy.

In my practice, the entire ultrasound study or a portion of the exam is performed in real time by the radiologist. I find this to be the most clinically accurate method, and it provides the most direct contact with the patient. Because I can see what I am feeling, it allows an "enhanced" physical examination of the area of concern identified by the patient or referring doctor.

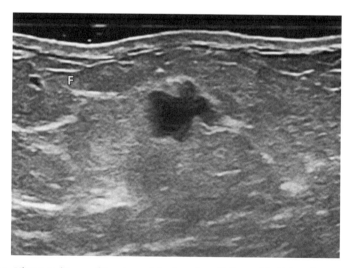

FIGURE 7.3 Ultrasound image. (Courtesy of the American College of Radiology.)

MAGNETIC RESONANCE IMAGING

Magnetic resonance imaging (MRI) uses extremely strong magnets (not harmful) to cause detectable changes in the tissue so that images can be produced; for breast tissue evaluation, a contrast dye (i.e., gadolinium) is also injected. The response of the tissue to the magnets, the timing of the pictures, and the amount of dye enhancement give information about the makeup of the tissue that can be useful in detecting cancers. See Figure 7.4.

MRI can be used as an adjunct to standard imaging such as mammography and ultrasound in the diagnostic setting or as a screening tool for high-risk patients. MRI is also useful for many patients who have had a recent diagnosis of breast cancer. As a preoperative assessment, it can help the surgeon plan the most appropriate approach to management by determining the full extent of the disease before the patient undergoes surgery. MRI also can be used to monitor the response to therapy in patients who receive chemotherapy before surgery to shrink the tumor. A shrinking lesion indicates that appropriate chemotherapy is being administered. Limited sequence MRI is being investigated and may prove to be a more cost effective and patient friendly alternative to full sequence MRI in the detection of breast cancer. Research is ongoing.

COMPUTER-AIDED DETECTION

A **computer-aided detection (CAD)** software program can be applied to film-screen or digital mammographic images. The software program contains data about mammographic findings that can indicate breast cancer, such as the presence of a small group of calcifications or a lesion with spiculations (i.e., thin, elongated pieces of tissue sticking out from the tumor mass). When the program scans the patient's film and detects

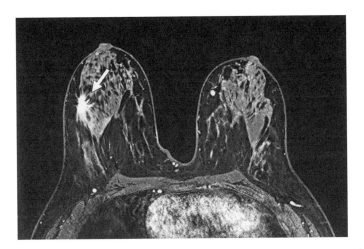

FIGURE 7.4 Magnetic resonance image. (Courtesy of the American College of Radiology.)

something that it has been programmed to find, it marks the location with an arrow or triangle, which alerts the radiologist to the problematic area.

The radiologist is responsible for determining the significance of the marked areas. Because CAD does not have the ability to compare old films or incorporate known surgical and biopsy histories, approximately 90% of the marks that it produces are *appropriately* ignored. On the other hand, CAD is most useful for detecting small clusters of calcifications that otherwise might have been missed or hidden in dense tissue. Although CAD aids the radiologist in lesion detection, it does not replace the interpretive skill of the radiologist, which incorporates many other factors in the assessment.

MOLECULAR IMAGING

Positron emission mammography (PEM): This specialized molecular imaging examination targets the increased uptake of glucose (i.e., sugar) by cancer cells. It employs a tracer to detect this activity in the cells. This technology can identify an area of cancer activity before it can be detected visually as a structure or mass with other imaging methods.

Breast-specific gamma imaging (BSGI): This specialized molecular imaging test uses a radioactive tracer that is injected into the patient. The radioactive material preferentially accumulates in tumors (i.e., cancers and some noncancerous tumors). A special gamma camera then detects the radioactive activity in the tumor cells and produces a picture. Like PEM, this is a less commonly used technology for breast imaging.

METHODS OF BIOPSY

Core needle biopsy: Core biopsy is the most common type of biopsy; it is performed in breast imaging because of its high yield of tissue and its accuracy. It is useful for laboratory evaluation of palpable and nonpalpable lesions ranging from mildly suspicious findings to obvious cancers. A hollow needle is used to retrieve a specimen that is about the size of a short spaghetti noodle (i.e., a "core" of tissue); this provides a generous amount of tissue for pathology evaluation. The accuracy is similar to that of surgical biopsy (see Chapter 12 and Fig. 7.5. Core biopsy can be performed under mammographic (sterotactic), ultrasound, or MRI guidance.

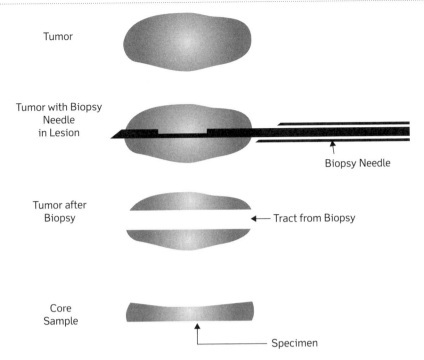

Tumor

Tumor with Biopsy
Needle
in Lesion

Biopsy Needle

Tumor after
Biopsy

← Tract from Biopsy

Core
Sample

Specimen

FIGURE 7.5 Needle biopsy sampling.

RADIOLOGY CONSULT

As a result of technologic advances and peer-reviewed research, more useful and more sensitive tests, less invasive ways to perform biopsies, more data on which to base decision making, and more efficient and accurate methods of approaching breast care are now available. We have never been in a better position in the entire history of medicine to deliver lifesaving breast imaging services with such a high level of quality as we can today. This fact is especially important because outside forces are actively trying to halt this trend and undermine its significance.

The Why

8

How It All Works: An Overview

A BIRD'S-EYE VIEW OF THE WHOLE PROCESS

MOST BREAST IMAGING centers are run as breast clinics. Patients are divided into two subgroups: screening and diagnostic. The two groups of patients are different in the manner in which their mammograms and other breast imaging examinations are performed and in how they are scheduled.

Screening patients have no symptoms (i.e., they are asymptomatic), or they have long-standing symptoms that are not worrisome. These women are scheduled routinely and receive examinations with standard mammographic views (usually two views of each breast) that typically are reviewed at a later time by the radiologist and usually are batch read for efficiency. Mammographic screening examinations usually take 10 to 15 minutes to perform.

For the general population, the current recommendation for screening mammography is annual imaging (i.e., every year) starting at age 40 years. High-risk women (i.e., those who are positive for a mutated *BRCA* gene, have a family history of breast cancer, or other factors) may require mammographic screening before age 40 or may benefit from the addition of screening **magnetic resonance imaging (MRI)** of the breast (highlighted terms are defined in the Glossary).

Diagnostic patients have symptoms of a breast abnormality, have been called back (i.e., recalled) after a screening study because of an abnormality found on the film, or have a clinical situation (e.g., prior lumpectomy for cancer) that requires special attention. The diagnostic study is a directed (i.e., problem-solving) examination that is used to address a specific issue. Comprehensive evaluation usually requires mammography and possibly **ultrasound**, breast MRI, and **biopsy**.

The diagnostic study is assessed by the radiologist at the same visit; this may take 30 minutes to 2 hours, depending on the complexity of the problem. During the evaluation

TABLE 8.1

Screening Versus Diagnostic Patients*

Screening Patients (Asymptomatic)	Diagnostic Patients (Symptomatic)
No breast-related symptoms	Lump or lumps, thickening, dimpling, skin changes, change in breast size
Chronic fibrocystic changes with no particular areas of concern	Fibrocystic changes with a particular area of concern
Diffuse (all over) breast pain with no specific area of concern	Focal breast pain in a specific spot or region
Contralateral breast in patient after mastectomy on the other side	
Nipple discharge (nonspontaneous, multiple ducts, white or nonbloody, bilateral) –At the discretion of referring physician	Nipple discharge (spontaneous, single duct, clear or bloody)
Asymptomatic patient with implants (requires implant displacement views)	Symptomatic patient with implants

Postlumpectomy (any subsequent mammogram after 5 years)
  –Depends on facility protocol
  –At the discretion of the referring physician
	After lumpectomy (at least the first mammogram after surgery, then annually for 5 years)
	  –At the discretion of the referring physician

After needle or excisional biopsy
  –All films after initial 6-month follow-up
	After needle or excisional biopsy
	  –If short-interval follow-up is recommended

Patient whose family or personal history necessitates earlier start of screening (usually 10 years before youngest age of diagnosis)	
	Follow-up of a previously identified abnormality (nonbiopsied lesions that are "probably benign" are usually followed for a total of 2 years)
	If patient or physician thinks the patient's symptoms or physical examination findings warrant diagnostic evaluation
	Any patient younger than age 40 years without a family history

*Lists do not include all clinical scenarios.

process, patients may receive a personal consultation with the radiologist, which usually involves a directed physical examination, a directed breast history, review of the findings, and explanation of the recommended disposition (i.e., what to do next as a result of the examination). In my practice, the radiologist sees all diagnostic patients, and the results and recommendations are explained to each patient at the time of evaluation.

The critical part of the breast imaging process is to ensure that the examination being performed (screening or diagnostic) fits the clinical situation and that the results are thoroughly assessed for the patient's specific situation. The **radiologic technologist** serves as the primary gatekeeper of this process and functions as an extension of the radiologist by reviewing the order, reviewing the medical history, and obtaining the patient's current medical status to ensure that the proper examination is being performed for the situation at hand. There must be a close working relationship between the technologist and the radiologist, with frequent exchange of information and reassessment of goals.

Table 8.1 gives an overview of common symptoms that determine whether a woman is a screening or a diagnostic patient.

The radiologist reviews the screening and diagnostic examinations to determine whether a finding on the image indicates possible (i.e., on the list of things to consider) or probable (i.e., the likely thing to consider) evidence of cancer. Standard protocols have been established based on research and experience that help to produce the most accurate results.

Chapters 9 and 10 discuss in more detail the signs, symptoms, and findings that are used to stratify patients into screening or diagnostic pathways; describe what a workup entails; and explain the specific factors that determine the decision-making tree.

RADIOLOGY CONSULT

Before an imaging examination is performed, it must be determined whether a woman is a candidate for a screening or a diagnostic evaluation. The goal is to fit the examination to the patient's history, symptoms (or absence of symptoms), and physical findings and to compare this profile with the doctor's order, which must support the history. The history taken by the technologist is an important part of the patient intake process. (No, they are not just being nosy!) Accurate history taking is paramount and helps to confirm that the patient is getting the examination that is appropriate for the clinical situation. Please be understanding if technologists seem to be nitpicking as they attempt to clarify a particular point or symptom. They are trying to gather pertinent information to guide the evaluation and assist the interpretation of the radiologic study.

9

How It All Works: The Screening Evaluation

SCREENING THE ASYMPTOMATIC POPULATION

AND SAVING LIVES

MAMMOGRAPHY IS BY far the most useful tool in screening for breast cancer. It is the only imaging modality that has been proven to decrease rates of **mortality** (death) for breast cancer (highlighted terms are defined in the Glossary). Screening patients are presumed by the radiologist to be asymptomatic (or to have chronic symptoms that are not worrisome) and to have negative findings on **self-breast examination (SBE**; breast check performed by the patient) and **clinical breast examination (CBE**; performed by the referring physician).

Box 9.1 lists chronic or nonsuspicious symptoms that may appropriately require a screening mammogram.

Screening the General Population

The current recommendation by the American College of Radiology (ACR), the Society of Breast Imaging (SBI), and the American College of Obstetrics and Gynecology (ACOG) for the general population is yearly screening mammography starting at age 40 years. Repeated annual examinations are emphasized to ensure detection of small abnormalities. Comparison of current and prior films makes subtle lesions much more perceptible to the radiologist, who can then be more confident in her interpretation.

Normal breast tissue can have a variety of appearances on a screening mammogram because the makeup of breast tissue can be predominantly fatty (gray), predominantly

BOX 9.1
SCREENING

Screening for Asymptomatic Patients

No breast-related symptoms

Chronic fibrocystic changes with no particular areas of concern

Diffuse (all over) breast pain with no specific area of concern

Contralateral breast in a patient after mastectomy on the other side

Nipple discharge (nonspontaneous, multiple ducts, white or nonbloody, bilateral)
    –At discretion of referring physician

Asymptomatic patients with implants (require implant displacement views)

Postlumpectomy (any subsequent mammogram after 5 years)
    –Depends on facility protocol
    –At the discretion of the referring physician

After needle or excisional biopsy
    –All films after initial 6-month follow-up

A patient whose family or personal history necessitates earlier start of screening
    (usually 10 years before youngest age of diagnosis)

*List does not include all clinical scenarios.

dense (white), or a mixture of the two. There are four main mammographic patterns, each of which can aid or limit image interpretation:

Fatty (0% to 24% dense tissue)
Average density (25% to 49% dense tissue)
Moderately dense (50% to 74% dense tissue)
Very dense (75% or dense tissue)

The breast tissue pattern is unique to each woman, just as her facial features are unique to her. As I tell my patients, "From year to year, you just have to continue to look like you." Figure 9.1 shows how these tissue patterns appear on mammogram images.

Figure 9.2 shows anatomy of the breast. Each year, radiologists look at and compare your current mammogram with previous images to ensure that you continue to "look like yourself." This comparison allows for more accurate image interpretation. For the radiologist, the stability of your pattern is a reassuring finding, and a new finding, even if subtle, can be more readily evident because it is a change from your normal pattern.

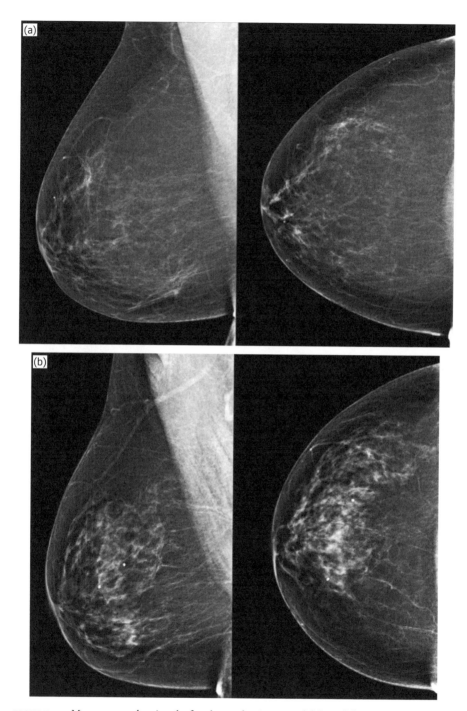

FIGURE 9.1 Mammogram showing the four breast density types. (a) fatty, (b) scattered or average, (c) heterogeneously or moderately dense, (d) extremely or very dense. (Courtesy of the American College of Radiology.)

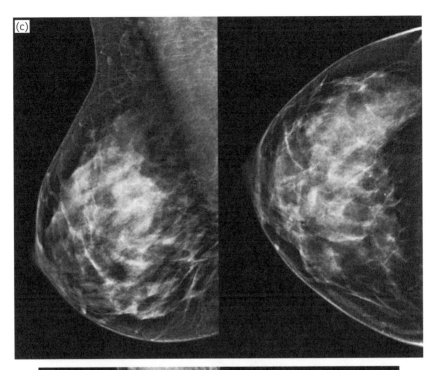

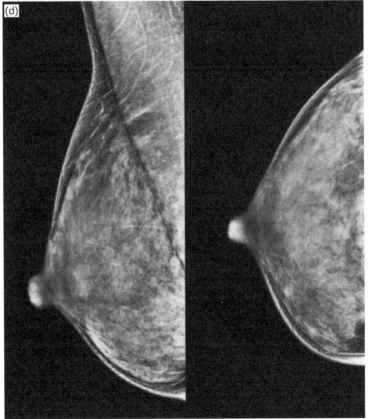

FIGURE 9.1 Continued.

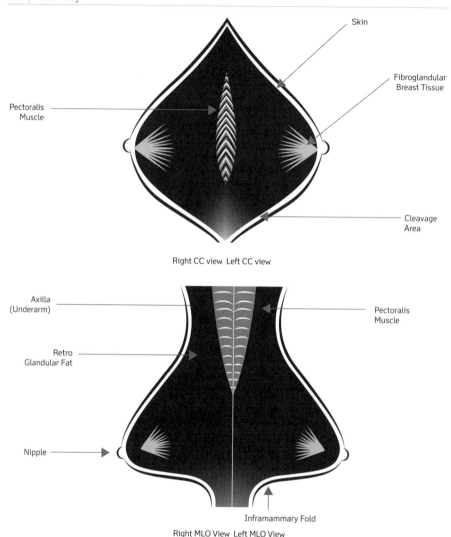

FIGURE 9.2 Anatomy of the breast on mammographic views.

How I Read Screening Mammograms

Image interpretation (now we are getting to the fun part!) is what the radiologist does to evaluate your films. Each radiologist has his or her own pattern of review, one that allows a consistent and structured evaluation process. Using this protocol, the radiologist can confirm that all areas of the film have been included in the review.

When interpreting a mammogram, my first order of business is to determine whether the film is good enough to read. I assess the technical adequacy of the images for positioning, compression, contrast, and artifacts because deficiencies in any of these areas can limit the interpretation of the film (i.e., limit my ability to detect a significant finding). Patient- related issues such as an inability to allow compression, limited mobility due to shoulder issues, kyphosis (i.e., bent spine), a fragile overall condition, or stroke, can hamper obtaining good images. When these limitations are noted by the technologist, I know that these are the "best films possible" for that particular patient, and I can proceed with the interpretation while being aware that there may be minor or even significant limitations to the review. If the limitation is significant, I usually write a note in the report so that the referring physician is aware of the situation.

After I have decided that the study is acceptable for reading, I go through a series of steps to interpret the film. First, I make a gestalt-like assessment, looking at the study as a whole for symmetry and obvious findings, and I compare it grossly with the previous studies, which I prefer to have displayed above the current study. I then review the current study in more detail by looking at each view of each breast in a specific sequence. I look for areas of concern that I need to address at the end of my review (Does this finding meet my criteria for normal, or does it need further evaluation?). I prefer to review the right and left cranial-caudal (CC) views side by side, followed by the right and left mediolateral oblique (MLO) views side by side. I then look at areas of special concern, such as the **retroareolar** region (i.e., behind the nipple), the medial aspect of the breast (i.e., cleavage area), the inframammary fold region (i.e., area at the bottom of the breast where it attaches to the abdominal wall), the retroglandular fat (i.e., area at the back of the breast at the junction of the breast tissue and the fatty tissue), and the **axilla** (i.e., armpit), looking at the lymph node region.

I assess the **tomographic** (three-dimensional) study as a rolling, real-time review while comparing it with the current two-dimensional (2-D) companion view. Because the 2-D image is digitally acquired, I can manipulate the image to optimize visualization of any areas of concern. By this time, I have usually made my assessment as to whether the examination result is negative (i.e., benign) or includes a finding that needs further evaluation.

At this point, I incorporate the **computer-aided detection (CAD)** software program in the interpretive process to see which areas of concern are identified by the computer. The software recognizes specific findings that it has been programmed to identify as suspicious based on how cancers can appear on the mammogram. I review what the CAD program has marked and determine whether these areas are concerning or can be discounted. The CAD program identifies many areas that may actually be normal tissue. It does not have the benefit of comparing to prior studies to determine that an area of concern is stable, and it is not able to incorporate the patient's history in the evaluation (e.g., knowing that an area of distortion is the result of a previous benign surgical biopsy and is of no concern).

The benefit of CAD is that it gives the radiologist multiple areas to review, reducing the likelihood that significant findings will be missed. CAD is particularly good for identifying small areas of calcification, which can be subtle and obscured in the background of dense tissue. After looking at the areas marked by the CAD program, I again review any concerning areas and make my final assessment.

Radiologists covet circumstances that optimize the interpretation of screening mammograms because of the sheer volume of images (over 50,000 per year at my facility). Protocols may include setting aside daily time slots for batch reading, thereby concentrating on only one type of examination at a time, and reading in a quiet place with few interruptions, where distraction is less likely. These conditions result in more accurate interpretations (i.e., less likelihood of missing important lesions) and more efficient workloads (i.e., greater number of films read in a specific time frame). The ultimate goal is to leave no stone unturned and no film unread!

What are we looking for? What findings are concerning? There are several categories of findings that can only be seen or are best seen mammographically:

1. Calcifications (which appear as white dots on a mammogram)
2. Mass or nodule
3. Increasing density (an area becoming more white, which reduces the ability to see through the tissue)
4. Architectural distortion (pulling of the tissue toward a central area)
5. New density (area of whiteness)
6. Subtle change in shape of an area (becoming more rounded and masslike, or with borders becoming irregular)
7. Global changes (i.e., diffuse change of the entire pattern)
8. Comparison with the other side (i.e., comparing left and right breasts)

Screening Women with Dense Breasts

Women with dense breast tissue account for about 50% of patients getting mammograms. The increased density of the breast tissue confers some increased risk of breast cancer relative to that of the general population. Supplemental (additional) testing is a current topic of discussion and debate, particularly because many states mandate notification about breast density for women receiving mammograms. However, I strongly emphasize the fact that screening mammography is the first line of testing for early detection of breast cancer in this group of patients, as in all women of screening age. Which additional tests are needed and at what intervals are debatable points, but the bottom line is that they all require, first and foremost, a screening mammogram.

As for any woman, I would optimize the mammogram for a woman with dense breast tissue to the greatest degree possible, for example by using **tomosynthesis (3-D mammography)** if possible. Screening ultrasound may have a role in this population, especially for those women with extremely dense tissue, who constitute 10% of the screened population. This topic is discussed further in Chapter 20.

Screening the High-Risk Population

As with the general population, the primary screening test for women with a high-risk profile is yearly screening mammography. Supplemental testing can be tailored to the patient and her specific risk profile.

Among women diagnosed with breast cancer, only 25% had known additional risk factors that significantly increased their risk above that of the general population. Most women vastly overestimate their lifetime risk of breast cancer, and their actual risk is much less than they perceive it to be. However, there are risk assessment models (e.g., Gail model, Tyrer-Cuzick model) that can determine a woman's risk and, based on the result, accurately put her into a high-risk group requiring additional testing.

A woman's history and other factors may put her into a high-risk category:

1. **Family history of breast cancer or ovarian cancer:** Assessment includes cancer in maternal and paternal relatives, primarily first-degree (e.g., mother, sister, daughter) and second-degree (e.g., grandmother, aunt, cousins) relatives. Red flags for susceptible families include cancer in members who are too young (i.e., premenopausal), in too many members (regardless of age), or in situations that are too unusual (e.g., male breast cancer). I usually recommend starting screening mammograms 10 years before the age of the youngest person diagnosed (e.g., if the patient's mother was diagnosed at age 40, she should start screening at age 30).

2. **Personal history of ovarian cancer:** Ovarian cancer is associated with a threefold to fourfold increased risk of breast cancer. Patients with a history of ovarian cancer should start annual mammography at the time of diagnosis, regardless of age, but not before age 25 years.

3. **Personal history of chest irradiation (i.e., mantle field irradiation):** These patients have a 4 to 75 times increased relative risk of breast cancer as a result of their mediastinal (midline chest) radiation. This is usually the result of treatment for Hodgkins lymphoma, and it is most significant for women treated between the ages of 10 and 30 years. Screening mammography should start 8 to 10 years after the radiation treatment, but not before age 25.

4. **Personal history of breast cancer:** Lumpectomy patients have a risk of recurrence (i.e., the cancer coming back) in the lumpectomy bed of 0.5% to 1.0% per year after surgery, with the highest risk during the first 5 to 7 years. I think it is reasonable for all lumpectomy patients to have diagnostic examinations during the first 5 years after treatment; after that, the referring doctor (usually the surgeon or oncologist) can determine whether the patient can return to a screening protocol or should continue diagnostic screenings indefinitely (which I personally prefer). Mastectomy patients require annual mammographic imaging of the unaffected breast.

5. **High-risk biopsy finding:** Lobular carcinoma in situ (LCIS), atypical ductal hyperplasia (ADH), and other high-risk pathologic findings from a surgical biopsy put patients at higher risk for development of breast cancer compared with the general population. The degree of additional risk is based on the specific diagnosis. Patients should have annual screening evaluations starting after the diagnosis or as directed by the referring physician (usually the surgeon), but not before age 25 years.

6. *BRCA* **positivity:** Patients with a mutated *BRCA* gene have a significantly higher lifetime risk of developing breast cancer compared with the general population. Because this risk can be as great as 40% to 80%, I recommend starting screening mammograms at age 25 years. Additional screening tests for breast cancer are also required. *BRCA*-positive patients and those patients with a greater than 25% lifetime risk as determined by a risk assessment tool benefit from screening **magnetic resonance imaging (MRI)** in addition to screening mammography. These patients should be in consultation with a genetics counselor because they are also at risk for ovarian cancer. There are other genetic conditions that can also predispose a woman to an increased risk of breast cancer. Panels of tests are available, and genetic counseling services are the best resource for accurate information about these tests and the implications of their results.

Several forms of supplemental imaging can be used for high-risk patients:

Tomosynthesis (i.e., 3-D mammography)
Screening ultrasound
Screening breast MRI (i.e., full sequence or abbreviated)
Contrast-enhanced mammography
Molecular imaging

Screening and Advanced Age

Because the medical literature supporting screening mammography does not include women older than 74 years of age, there are no objective data to support screening mammography for this group. However, there is also no evidence to indicate that screening mammography would not continue to provide the same benefits after age 74 as it did previously.

The decision to screen any woman should also be based on comorbid conditions (i.e., associated illnesses or disorders) and the patient's overall health. Certain younger patients with severe comorbid disease and those who cannot cooperate with the examination well enough for it to be performed properly (i.e., women with mental or physical limitations) should not be getting screening mammograms. Even if cancer were diagnosed in one of these patients, she could not tolerate the treatment or ongoing care needed. If a patient older than age 75 is expected to live for another 5 years or longer, screening mammography seems reasonable. I do not refuse screening mammography to a patient based on advanced age, and I believe that it is indicated for older women in whom a detected breast cancer would be treated.

RADIOLOGY CONSULT

The two biggest risk factors for breast cancer are gender (being female) and age (getting older); 75% of women diagnosed with breast cancer have no known family history or risk factors. These facts justify screening the general population of women who are at average risk. Annual screening of these women starting at age 40 years saves the most lives. Data also support earlier or increased surveillance for identified high-risk populations, such as women with a strong family history of cancer or *BRCA* gene positivity. However, there are no known findings that would put a woman into a low-risk category and eliminate the need to be screened—so we cannot take any group off the screening list yet.

10

How It All Works: The Diagnostic Evaluation

SYMPTOMATIC PATIENTS AND THE JOURNEY TO

THE CORRECT DIAGNOSIS

THE DIAGNOSTIC PROCESS involving a breast-related problem is easily one of the most anxiety-provoking situations in a woman's health care experience. The relative lack of understanding about this process and the fear of being told that you may have breast cancer often interfere with your ability to participate effectively in the process and the radiology staff's ability to optimally or efficiently perform the evaluation. And believe me, it is no small feat to successfully guide a tearful, anxious woman—now placed in an unfamiliar setting where she may feel vulnerable—through a complete diagnostic evaluation with everyone's nerves still intact!

Unlike the screening process, the diagnostic evaluation is a problem-solving endeavor. The workup requires more time than a screening evaluation as well as direct, active supervision by a **radiologist** (highlighted terms are defined in the Glossary). The radiologist reviews the films to ensure that the examination is appropriately performed and that all questionable findings are thoroughly analyzed. To assist you in understanding this type of evaluation, this chapter outlines the most frequent types of diagnostic scenarios so that you can easily identify your situation or symptom and "follow along" with the evaluation process.

The Basics

The standard studies included in a diagnostic evaluation are **mammography**, **ultrasound**, and, increasingly, breast **magnetic resonance imaging (MRI)**. In addition, the radiologist may personally perform a directed history and physical examination or perform the ultrasound in real time to better evaluate the findings and clarify the data in your case.

Based on the incidence of breast cancer and the inherent risks in particular age groups, certain basic guidelines are used when proceeding with a diagnostic evaluation. Although the exact age categories are somewhat arbitrary, the guidelines should be consistent within a given facility. At my institution, the protocol is as follows:

1. Women younger than 25 years of age
   a. Ultrasound only (most surgeons are willing to go to surgery based on the ultrasound findings alone)
   b. Mammography only in extraordinary circumstances (limited views as directed by the radiologist)
2. Women between 25 and 29 years of age
   a. Ultrasound first
   b. Mammography as indicated by radiologist
3. Women 30 years of age or older
   a. Mammography as the first line of evaluation
   b. Ultrasound as indicated

These age criteria may be adjusted if the profile indicates increased risk, such as strong family history or gene positivity. For example, if you are 27 years old and present with a lump but your mother was diagnosed with breast cancer at age 33, a bilateral mammogram will be performed, and bilateral survey ultrasound including directed ultrasound of the lump, to provide thorough screening for breast cancer in addition to addressing the issue of your lump. In general, the lower age limit for mammography is 25 years even in the context of a high-risk profile.

INDICATIONS FOR A DIAGNOSTIC EVALUATION

In addition to the basic question—"Is there evidence of breast cancer?"—a diagnostic evaluation of the breasts may be performed for many other reasons (Box 10.1). For example, there may be a specific question (or problem) that needs to be addressed. The following specific situations may occur:

1. You are **recalled** after a screening mammogram because of
   A. Technical recall
   B. Calcifications
   C. Well defined nodule or mass

BOX 10.1
DIAGNOSTIC SYMPTOMS*

Diagnostic (Symptomatic)

A lump or lumps, thickening, dimpling, skin changes, or change in breast size

Fibrocystic changes with a particular area of concern

Focal breast pain (in a specific spot or region)

Nipple discharge (spontaneous, single duct, clear or bloody)

Symptomatic patients with implants

Previous lumpectomy (at least the first mammogram after surgery, then annually for 5 years)

    –at the discretion of the referring physician

Previous needle or excisional biopsy

    –if short-interval follow-up is recommended)

Follow-up of a previously identified abnormality (nonbiopsied lesions that are "probably benign" are usually followed for a total of 2 years)

If the patient or the physician believes that the patient's symptoms or physical examination findings warrant diagnostic evaluation

Any patient younger than 40 years of age without a family history

---

*List does not include all clinical scenarios.

    D. Poorly defined nodule or mass
    E. Asymmetric density
    F. Architectural distortion
2. You are **symptomatic** or have a **physical finding** and present with
    A. Palpable abnormality (lump, mass, or thickening)
    B. Pain and/or swelling
    C. Nipple discharge
    D. Skin changes
    E. Change in breast size
3. You have a **history** that requires special attention, such as
    A. Surveillance of a previous lesion found to be "probably benign"
    B. Follow-up of a previous benign biopsy result
    C. History of breast cancer, especially lumpectomy
    D. Incidental breast finding seen on a non-breast study
    E. Search for the primary tumor in a patient with metastatic disease

Each of these scenarios is discussed in the expanded discussion section of this chapter.

At the conclusion of a typical diagnostic evaluation, the radiologist makes a determination as to the degree of suspicion of breast cancer (or lack thereof) and also addresses the specific reason the evaluation was initiated. For example, Are the calcifications suspicious and require biopsy? Is the lump that you palpate a benign cyst? Is the assessment incomplete with additional imaging needed to gather more information? Would old films help to clarify a finding's significance?

REPORTING CATEGORIES

As required by the **Mammography Quality Standards Act of 1992 (MQSA)**, all breast evaluations that include mammography (and increasingly, by convention, all other breast imaging studies) should designate a final Category (see Topics in Breast Imaging: Terms About Conclusions and Recommendations) that reflects the overall assessment and conveys to the referring physician the actions needed as a result of the recommendation.

In the diagnostic scenario, the Breast Imaging Reporting and Data System (BIRADS) mandates the following **Categories** (see Topics in Breast Imaging and the Glossary at the end of this book).

Category 0: Incomplete Evaluation

This category may be reported for two reasons. A report of **Category 0: Incomplete Evaluation—Additional Imaging Needed** means additional workup is needed to determine if a finding is suspicious or not. This is commonly used when a finding is seen on a screening mammogram and the radiologist wants to investigate the finding further to determine it's level of suspicion. This work up may include diagnositic mammography and ultrasound. Additionally, but less frequently at the end of a standard diagnositic evaluation it may be concluded that an MRI or other imaging study might add helpful information to increase the radiologist's ability to make an appropriate recommendation. For example, a **lesion** may be persistent but vague on the mammogram, not seen on ultrasound, and not palpable; in such a case, breast MRI may confirm that the lesion is a real and suspicious finding that warrants biopsy rather than follow-up.

A report of **Category 0: Incomplete Evaluation—Awaiting Prior Films** may be given if imaging studies or biopsies were performed in the past but the reports and/or films were not available at the time of the diagnostic evaluation. If this information can be retrieved and could reasonably change the radiologist's recommendation, it is usually worth delaying the final report until the information is available. If the information does not become available, the final recommendation will be based on the available data (even if known to be limited). For example, a nodule may be seen sonographically (i.e., by ultrasound) and would ordinarily warrant biopsy, but the patient reports that she had a previous benign needle biopsy in the same general area at a facility in another state 5 years ago. Is it the same lesion? Has it been previously biopsied, or is it a new lesion located in the same area of the breast? Without the old films, it is impossible to be sure, and a repeat biopsy of the lesion may be (rightfully) performed for tissue confirmation because of the lack of supporting confirmatory information.

Category 1: Negative

A report of **Category 1: Negative** means that there is no evidence of malignancy; routine imaging is recommended. However, there is one caveat to this category in the context of a diagnostic evaluation: If the evaluation was initiated because of a highly supicious palpable abnormality, a negative imaging evaluation does not mean that no further evaluation is needed, just that the images reveal no suspicious findings. This is an uncommon occurance, but in this situation, I usually add the following statement: "Clinical follow-up as per referring physician. As with any palpable abnormality, if there is persistent or increasing concern, consider surgical consultation for second opinion even in the context of benign imaging." This is necessary because a discrete or concerning clinical finding should not be ignored just because the imaging studies are (legitimately) unremarkable.

Category 2: Benign

A report of **Category 2: Benign** means that a finding may have been observed but is believed to have no likelihood of malignancy; routine imaging is recommended. If the lesion is palpable, I also add the same statement as for Category 1 regarding clinical follow-up.

Category 3: Probably Benign

A report of **Category 3: Probably Benign** means that a finding was identified but is believed to have an extremely low likelihood of malignancy (less than 2%). Short-interval follow-up is recommended, which usually means follow-up at 6 months with mammography, ultrasound, or even MRI. A shorter interval may be needed if the findings are believed to be infectious or trauma related and are expected to change more quickly (e.g., in response to treatment or healing; see Chapter 11).

Category 4: Suspicious

A report of **Category 4: Suspicious** means that cancer is a *possibility*. However, there are gradations in the level of concern for malignancy (see Topics in Breast Imaging: Terms About Imaging Findings at the end of this book). For example, the possibility of malignancy may be mild (i.e., cancer is possible but not highly expected), or it may be moderate (i.e., cancer is likely but not definite). Biopsy is warranted for most Category 4 lesions.

Category 5: Highly Suspicious

A report of **Category 5: Highly Suspicious** means that cancer is *probable*. The lesion is very likely to be malignant based on its characteristics and therefore definitely warrants biopsy.

Category 6: Known Malignancy

A report of **Category 6: Known Malignancy** may be given if the evaluation undertaken to investigate other areas of the breast in a patient with biopsy-proven cancer to determine the extent of disease, to monitor a cancer in a patient who has refused treatment to assess for interval growth and spread, or as a follow-up examination in someone who has received neoadjuvant (presurgical) chemotherapy to assess the response of the **tumor** to the therapy.

If the final conclusion from your evaluation is a recommendation for biopsy, don't panic—refer to Chapter 12.

Review of the Diagnostic Evaluation Process

It is now time to begin our review of the diagnostic evaluation process. First, each category is discussed in general terms, and then the individual topics are explored in more detail. Each section has an *"Is This You?"* sample case scenario to demonstrate how the particular topic might be addressed in a clinical setting and to give you a real-life feel for the material. Each also includes a *Radiology Consult* section to provide pointed advice on the topic from the viewpoint of the interpreting radiologist. My goal is that by the end of this review you will have a greater understanding of and lesser anxiety about the whole process. So, let's get started.

I. YOU ARE RECALLED AFTER A SCREENING MAMMOGRAM

A recall, or callback, occurs when you have had a screening mammogram and are requested to return for additional imaging because an **abnormality** has been noted by the interpreting radiologist and further clarification is needed in order to make a final recommendation. Recall rates vary depending on the experience and training of the radiologist, the equipment used, and the community standards of the area in which the radiologist practices. Acceptable rates range from 8% to 12%. In other words, if a radiologist reads 1000 screening mammograms, approximately 80 to 120 women will be called back for additional imaging. (The typical incidence of cancer in a screening population is 3 to 6 cases per 1000).

Recall rates are usually higher in a previously unscreened population (i.e., women getting their first or **baseline** examination), compared with previously screened populations. This occurs because the unscreened population has no prior imaging that the radiologist can use to compare the stability of findings or of your distinct parenchymal pattern (i.e., features that make your breast pattern unique to you). Therefore, some of the findings may need to be evaluated or biopsy may need to be performed to confirm their benign nature.

In the callback scenario, it is presumed that you are asymptomatic and have negative findings on **self-breast examination (SBE)** and **clinical breast examination (CBE)**. In this setting, you have presented for a screening mammogram, and on review of the films, the radiologist has detected a finding that requires further evaluation. Additional mammography, ultrasound, MRI, or other imaging may be required to determine the level of suspicion—in other words, a **workup** is needed.

A callback does not necessarily mean that the lesion is suspicious, just that insufficient information is available based on the initial screening study and more information can be gained with additional testing through a diagnostic examination. Many times, the lack of prior films or history necessitates a recall because there is a finding that cannot be confirmed to be stable—so bring your old films with you, please! In a properly screened population, a change observed by comparing the current and prior examinations may result in a callback.

Now let's review the common findings that necessitate recalls and discuss what determines the types of studies needed to address the finding or concern. Included in the discussion are technical recalls as well as recalls for calcifications, well defined and poorly defined nodules and masses, asymmetric densities, and architectural distortion.

A. Technical Recall

A technical recall is a callback based on technical factors that have led to a poorly performed study or portion of a study. Examples are motion, poor positioning, and artifacts. These should not be common, but they are an unavoidable part of the process given the ability of the patient to cooperate with the examination, and sometimes the conditions under which the examination is performed. The supervising technologist closely monitors the frequency of these callbacks to identify any processing or equipment deficiencies and decides whether particular technologists need additional training. Even outstanding technologists have technical callbacks occasionally—life's not perfect. The patient is called or receives a letter requesting that she return for repeat imaging to complete the initial screening examination for the purpose of making the study adequate for interpretation.

Although a technical recall is not a true diagnostic evaluation, it is usually treated as such and performed when a radiologist is available. That way, the radiologist can review the films, first for technical adequacy (Are the images good enough to read?) and then for actual interpretation of the films for abnormalities (Are there findings that need further evaluation?). This ensures that if there is a truly suspicious finding, you will not need to make yet another trip to the facility. The repeat (or technical recall) portion of an examination should be performed at no additional charge to you because it merely completes the screening examination. If additional imaging is needed because an abnormality is found, the diagnostic workup should proceed as with any other callback (see later discussion).

Admit it: Some of you become annoyed about such recalls, even hostile. I would suggest, however, that you should actually be glad that the interpreting radiologist is diligent enough to require the best films possible for your assessment. The request for repeat images shows (1) that the radiologist is paying attention to the technical aspects of the film and (2) that the radiologist will not accept substandard films for your evaluation. Please view this as a good thing.

The following are common reasons for technical recalls:

Motion (most common reason)
Suboptimal positioning (not enough breast tissue on the film)
Suboptimal compression (limited ability to "see through" the tissue because the
    tissue is not separated out enough)
Artifacts (e.g., dust, fingerprints, hair, deodorant)

"IS THIS YOU?" SAMPLE CASE SCENARIO

A 49-year-old woman presents for her **screening mammogram**. She is premenopausal, and the examination is being performed one week before the expected onset of her menstrual period, so her breasts are somewhat tender.

The four routine views are obtained—**cranial-caudal (CC)** and **mediolateral-oblique (MLO)** views of each breast. The technologist checks the films, and they appear technically adequate.

The patient is discharged from the breast center and told that the films will be read the following day, with a report sent to her doctor soon thereafter. In addition, a "lay letter" will be sent to her directly to notify her of the results, as required by MQSA.

In the process of reviewing the patient's films, the radiologist notices that the right MLO view has some motion. This is evident because of the blurry and smudgy appearance of the parenchymal lines in this view compared with the other views—the image is not as sharp. This type of finding is seen best by the radiologist, who reads the films in a dark room and has the tools that can be used for interpretation (e.g., computer manipulation and magnification). The motion has probably occurred because the patient inadvertently pulled back during the examination due to tenderness of the breast.

A report is generated stating that the right mammogram is incomplete for technical reasons and a repeat right MLO view is required to complete the evaluation. The examination is reported as **Category 0: Incomplete Evaluation—Additional Imaging Needed**.

The patient is called by the breast center staff, and a repeat right MLO (**diagnostic right mammogram**) is scheduled for the following day.

The radiologist reviews the repeat MLO film for technical adequacy, finds it acceptable, and then interprets it in conjunction with the initial films. Calcifications that were not visible initially are seen on today's film, but they are clearly vascular in origin (i.e., located in the wall of a vessel) and not concerning.

The radiologist's final assessment is that the patient has no findings suspicious for malignancy and can return to annual imaging. The examination is reported as a **Category 2: Benign**. This is communicated to the patient via the performing technologist or the radiologist, and the patient is discharged.

RADIOLOGY CONSULT

The point in a woman's menstrual cycle at which her breasts are most tender is usually the week before the start of her period. If you are someone who has tenderness associated with your cycle, schedule your mammogram during the week after the start of your period, if possible, to minimize tenderness. This will allow better compression, better positioning, and a decreased likelihood of motion on your part due to breast tenderness.

B. Calcifications

Calcifications are very common and on some days could be considered the bane of my existence! They are common, common, and—did I mention?—common! Calcifications may result from any number of processes within the breast, the vast majority of which are benign and normal. They are not believed to be associated with nutritional intake of calcium supplements or calcium in your diet. Calcifications may also be the seen in association with fibrocystic changes in the breast, within benign tumors, as a result of trauma, or as a result of the healing process after surgery or radiation therapy.

However, and more importantly, calcifications can also be the earliest imaging manifestation of malignancy. The good news is that when such malignancies are diagnosed, they are frequently in an early, potentially curable stage. The challenge lies in trying to determine which calcifications are benign and can be left alone, which require recall, and which require biopsy because they may represent malignancy. The goal for the radiologist is to have no missed cancers and to capture all of the true cancers in the group of women who are called back and biopsied.

It is important to remember that there is definitely overlap in the imaging appearance of some benign processes (e.g., sclerosing adenosis) when compared with early-stage cancers. Two groups of calcifications can look identical on mammography even if one is cancer and the other is not. However, benign conditions are much more common than cancer, so the odds are in your favor. What is significant is the definitive result of your individual finding, not just a general statistic: If you are the one with the cancer, then who cares if there is a 70% statistical likelihood of benign pathology based on the imaging appearance?

Furthermore, if radiologists waited until all cancers showed the obvious characteristics of cancer, the **specificity** of our findings (i.e., when we call it cancer, it is truly cancer) would be great, but this would not be very helpful in decreasing mortality from breast cancer because in many cases we would have waited too long and the cancer would be too advanced to make a cure reasonably possible. Therefore, inherent in the process of evaluating calcifications is the knowledge that to find the early cancers we *must* biopsy some benign calcifications, because they can be indistinguishable from cancer based on imaging appearance alone.

For the most part, follow-up of calcifications has not been found to be very useful because stability of calcifications does not exclude malignancy. Calcifications can be stable for a long time (as an early-stage process) and then develop obvious characteristics of cancer (now possibly later-stage disease) after years of follow-up. If the calcifications are suspicious, they should be biopsied. **Stereotactically guided** needle biopsy has led to a remarkable advance in women's health care over the last 20 years; it provides an easy and safe method of biopsy in an outpatient setting.

Mammography is *the* definitive study used to evaluate calcifications. It is our first-line study to get detailed information about them. Ultrasound has become increasingly more useful in the evaluation of some types of calcifications, particularly if there is a density associated with them. Ultrasound may locate the invasive component of the process and may be used to guide biopsy of the area in some cases. MRI is of no practical use in the initial assessment of calcifications.

The mammographic evaluation of calcifications should always include true lateral (90-degree) imaging to assess for so-called milk of calcium (i.e., calcium within the fluid medium of a cyst); if this is diagnosed, the lesion is clearly benign and does not require biopsy. To explain: Imagine that a cyst is a water balloon with calcium particles floating within the water medium. The concept is that the calcium is heavier than the other fluid and will settle to the bottom of the cyst. If pictured from the side (horizontal plane), the calcium will show up on the mammogram as a semicircle or white line as in the bottom of a teacup (i.e., a layer of calcium has settled on the cyst floor), confirming that it is within a fluid solution (Fig. 10.1). Although the cyst itself is not seen, its presence is inferred from the presence of the milk of calcium. A confirmed cyst means, in effect, no cancer. Great!

Magnification views are frequently needed because the calcifications of interest are small. The magnified views assist the radiologist in visual assessment of the process and assessment of shape and other characteristics of the calcifications.

The following characteristics of calcifications are worrisome and may require biopsy (Fig. 10.2):

1) Cyst

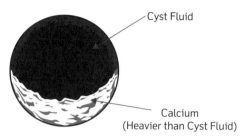

Cyst Fluid

Calcium
(Heavier than Cyst Fluid)

2) Mammogram (true lateral)

Head

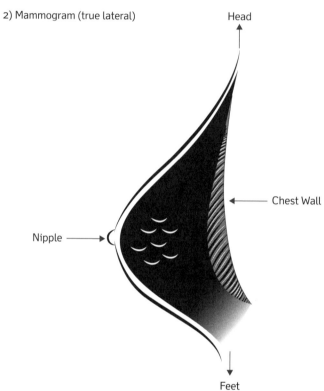

Chest Wall

Nipple

Feet

FIGURE 10.1 Benign milk of calcium.

Pleomorphic
(Different Shapes
and Sizes; Crushed
Glass Appearance)

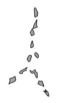

Linear Distribution
(Forming a Line)

Grouped/Clustered

FIGURE 10.2 Suspicious calcifications.

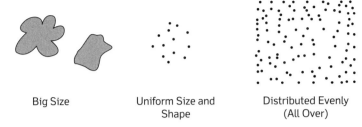

Big Size   Uniform Size and   Distributed Evenly
                  Shape   (All Over)

FIGURE 10.3 Favorable calcifications.

Clustered (tightly grouped together)
Pleomorphic (different shapes and sizes;—they don't look like their neighbor)
Linear distribution (forming a line or "ductal" pattern)
New
Increasing in number

The following characteristics of calcifications are not worrisome and do not require biopsy (Fig. 10.3):

Milk of calcium
Large, coarse, "popcorn" appearance
Smooth, round, "pearl-like" shape
Rim calcifications (i.e., at the periphery of a lesion)
Scattered or loosely grouped distribution

"IS THIS YOU?" SAMPLE CASE SCENARIO

A 63-year-old woman presents for her **screening mammogram** and is found to have new calcifications in the upper inner quadrant of the left breast (LUIQ). Her examination is reported as a **Category 0: Incomplete Evaluation—Additional Imaging Needed.**

The patient returns for a unilateral left **diagnostic mammogram** 2 days later. At that time, a full true lateral (90-degree) view and spot magnification views in the CC and lateral projections are obtained to better visualize and assess the calcifications in the LUIQ.

The additional views reveal the calcifications to be clustered and pleomorphic (i.e., having different sizes and shapes). They do not layer and therefore are not milk of calcium. The calcifications are believed to be suspicious enough to warrant biopsy. The evaluation is reported as **Category 4: Suspicious. A stereotactically (mammogram) guided needle biopsy** is recommended.

The films are reviewed with the patient, and the recommendation is discussed with her at the time of the evaluation. She is scheduled for **stereotactically guided needle biopsy**.

A week later, the patient returns for the **stereotactic biopsy**. The calcifications are targeted and are confirmed by the specimen radiograph (i.e., x-ray examination of the tissue that was removed) to be adequately sampled, meaning that many calcifications are visible on the film (see Chapter 11). The patient tolerates the procedure well, and there are no complications. The specimens are sent to the pathology department, where they are analyzed and interpreted by the pathologist.

Four days later, a final pathology report is available. The evaluation has revealed a diagnosis of malignancy: **ductal carcinoma in situ (DCIS)**.

RADIOLOGY CONSULT

Routine annual mammograms give the radiologist the best opportunity to find subtle, small changes on your film. Finding a malignant lesion at the earliest possible time—as soon as it becomes visually detectible—may catch it at an earlier stage of disease, and that usually correlates with improved survival. Early detection is the key.

C. Well-Defined Nodule or Mass

If you are called back because a **well-defined** (i.e., with a crisp, sharp border) **nodule or mass** was seen on screening mammography and its location is known or clear based on the mammogram (i.e., seen in both views), the diagnostic evaluation can start directly with ultrasound. This will determine whether the lesion is a cyst or is solid. If the lesion is a cyst, no further work-up is needed, and you can return to your routine screening protocol. If the lesion is probably—but not definitively—a cyst, then ultrasound guided aspiration may be performed to confirm this diagnosis. If the lesion is solid, then the characteristics of the lesion will be assessed by ultrasound to determine whether biopsy is warranted.

In this scenario, because you presented for a screening mammogram, it is presumed that you are asymptomatic and the SBE and CBE are negative—that is, the lesion is not **palpable** and is not causing any clinical symptoms. Therefore, if certain criteria are met, the lesion can be considered "probably benign" and routine imaging surveillance can be recommended rather than biopsy. However, if the lesion is new, is increasing, or does not meet the criteria for surveillance, biopsy would be required.

Occasionally, a slow-growing (usually well-differentiated and low-grade) cancer manifests as a well-defined nodule or mass. In such cases, it may simulate a benign or favorable process. This underscores the importance of annual mammograms, in that changes can be subtle and the only finding alerting the radiologist to the need for biopsy may be the change from a prior mammogram or imaging study.

The following characteristics of a well-defined solid nodule are favorable (Fig. 10.4):

Round or oval shape (i.e., just "hanging out," not invading the surrounding tissues)
Homogeneous ("color" is similar throughout the lesion)
Good through-transmission (i.e., ultrasound easily penetrates the lesion, inferring that it is not very dense)

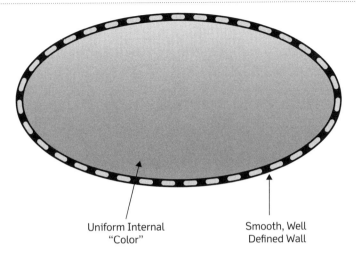

FIGURE 10.4 Characteristic appearance of a favorable solid mass.

"IS THIS YOU?" SAMPLE CASE SCENARIO

A 57-year-old postmenopausal woman presents for her annual **screening mammogram** and is found to have a new **retroareolar** (behind the nipple) nodule on the left breast and an increasing nodule in the upper outer quadrant of the right breast (RUOQ). She is asymptomatic and is taking hormone replacement therapy (HRT).

Her examination is reported as **Category 0: Incomplete Evaluation—Additional Imaging Needed.**

She returns one week later for a directed **ultrasound** examination of both nodules.

Ultrasound reveals that both the left retroareolar nodule and the RUOQ nodule represent simple cysts (Fig. 10.5). The patient is without symptoms related to the cysts, so **cyst aspiration** is deferred.

Her evaluation is reported as **Category 2: Benign,** and she can return to annual imaging.

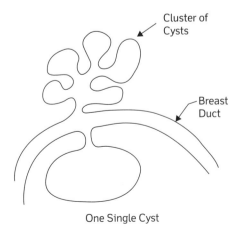

FIGURE 10.5 Characteristic appearance of a cyst and a cluster of cysts.

> **RADIOLOGY CONSULT**
>
> Cysts can occur spontaneously, but they are also a common side effect of HRT. Cysts are not a reason to change or discontinue your hormone regimen if they are confirmed to be cysts. Confirmed cysts do not require intervention if they are asymptomatic (not causing pain or nonpalpable). A cyst that is symptomatic can be aspirated if the pain is significant (and aspiration will help relieve the pain) or if it bothers the patient that the cyst is palpable. Benign cysts are not cancer and do not turn into cancer—so if they don't bother you, they don't bother me. Aspiration is not needed, and you can return to annual mammographic screening.

D. Poorly Defined Nodule or Mass

If you are called back because of a **poorly defined nodule or mass** (Fig. 10.6), the diagnostic evaluation will usually start with additional mammographic films. This is done to

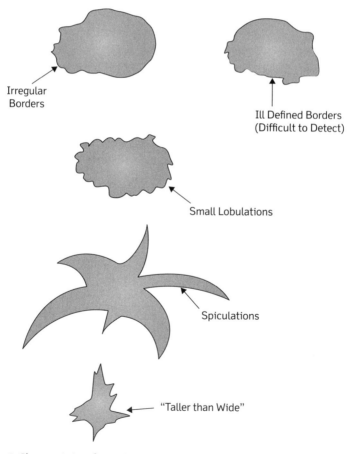

FIGURE 10.6 Characteristics of a suspicious mass.

further evaluate the border of the lesion and to assess for other associated findings such as calcifications. Your workup will likely include some sort of focal compression views that in essence push the surrounding tissue out of the way or thin the tissue to make it easier to see through to the mass itself. Are the borders of the mass really poorly defined, or were they just obscured by overlying tissue? Are there calcifications associated with the lesion? Are the calcifications located only within the lesion, or are they now evident over a larger area? Are other lesions now evident in the surrounding tissue? All of these questions can be addressed with these additional mammographic images. If your initial mammogram was a two-dimensional (2-D) study, additional **tomographic** (3-D) imaging is usually very helpful in this instance. If your initial screening mammogram was 3-D, then you may require only ultrasound evaluation at callback because the amount of mammographic information needed to make an assessment has already been acquired on the 3-D study.

Once the mammographic evaluation is complete, the assessment proceeds to ultrasound to further characterize the lesion and to determine whether ultrasound can be used for guidance if biopsy is warranted. The determination of whether biopsy is needed can usually be made based on the findings from these two types of examinations. If a lesion is persistent and is confirmed to have ill-defined or poorly defined borders, then image guided needle biopsy is likely to be recommended.

"IS THIS YOU?" SAMPLE CASE SCENARIO

A 75-year-old woman presents for her **screening mammogram**, and an irregular density is noted in the inferior aspect of the left breast. Her examination is reported as **Category 0: Incomplete Evaluation—Additional Imaging Needed**.

The patient's return visit to the breast center is delayed because she is the sole caretaker for her husband who recently suffered a stroke. One month later, she is able to get a friend to care for her husband for the day and returns for a **diagnostic left mammogram** and **left breast ultrasound** study.

The **diagnostic mammogram** consists of a true lateral (90-degree) view and spot compression views of the lesion in the CC and MLO projections. The lesion is confirmed to be real and the borders of the lesion to be indeed irregular.

Sonography (ultrasound) reveals the lesion to be solid and angulated. Significant shadowing and prominent vascularity within the lesion are also noted.

On directed physical examination (i.e., knowing the exact location while scanning with the ultrasound), the radiologist finds that the lesion is vaguely palpable and is firm, grainy, and fixed.

The lesion is believed to be clinically, mammographically, and sonographically consistent with a primary breast malignancy, and biopsy is recommended. The evaluation is reported as **Category 5: Highly Suspicious**, and biopsy is recommended.

Because of the patient's social situation and her limited ability to return within a reasonable time frame, an **ultrasound-guided core needle biopsy** is performed on the same day. The tissue is sent to the pathology department for analysis and interpretation by the pathologist.

Two days later, the pathology report is available. It confirms the diagnosis of malignancy: **invasive ductal carcinoma (IDC)**, grade 3.

RADIOLOGY CONSULT

Real-time evaluation with ultrasound can augment the physical examination of the breast. Knowing exactly where to feel and concentrating on an area based on the ultrasound findings can greatly enhance the CBE performed by the ultrasound technologist or the radiologist. Ultrasound technologists should be encouraged to use this tool in their assessments and to report their findings to the radiologist. This is a typical experience in my practice because radiologists perform the vast majority of the ultrasound examinations themselves. This adds an additional level of confidence in the recommendation being made. It allows for interaction with the patient, gives me an opportunity to explain the findings and recommendations, and also gives the patient the opportunity to ask questions.

E. Asymmetric Density

I have been known to say that although breasts may look the same on the outside, they are usually not "twins" on the inside. This means that it is common to have asymmetries and differences in the mammographic appearance of one breast compared with the other (Fig. 10.7). That being said, symmetry (equal distribution in both breasts) is one of the findings that radiologists use to determine whether a finding is concerning. In general, findings that are symmetric are benign; it is rare to have cancers that are both **synchronous** (i.e., occurring at the same time) and mirror images of each other (i.e., at same place in both breasts). Therefore, symmetry is generally a good thing. Asymmetry, although it can be normal, may indicate an abnormality, especially if it is developing over time and does not represent your established parenchymal pattern.

On a baseline examination, an area of asymmetry may stand out and require additional workup simply because there is no prior study with which to document stability. If a change from a prior mammogram is found, it may represent (1) changes in technique and positioning, (2) overlapping tissue or structures, or (3) the true development of a mass (which could indicate the presence of a malignancy). The most common reason for real but nonmalignant changes in the density of breast tissue is hormonal influences, especially HRT.

The purpose of the diagnostic evaluation for **asymmetric density** is to determine, first and foremost, whether this is a real lesion. The diagnostic evaluation, then, starts

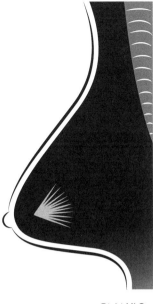
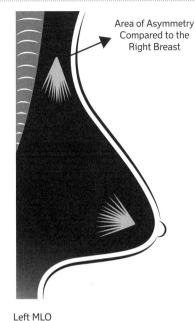

Area of Asymmetry
Compared to the
Right Breast

Right MLO   Left MLO

FIGURE 10.7 Asymmetry.

with additional mammographic imaging. These special views are performed to determine whether technique, positioning, or overlapping tissues are the cause of the perceived density. The area of interest is imaged from various directions, and compression views are obtained to spread out the tissue for better visualization. If the lesion is not real, it will appear less conspicuous (less visually evident) on additional imaging or may go away completely (efface). A real lesion is likely to become more obvious or more conspicuous with additional imaging because the surrounding and obscuring normal tissue has been pushed out of the way. If the lesion persists or if the radiologist thinks that it will be helpful in evaluating the finding, an ultrasound examination will be performed. It provides additional data to either confirm or oppose a mammographic opinion.

Another scenario occurs when the lesion effaces and no longer persists as a suspicious abnormality; in that case, no further workup is needed, and you can return to routine imaging. Also, if the lesion persists but has an appearance most consistent with asymmetry of normal tissue, then, based on the level of certainty, the radiologist may place you back into a routine screening protocol or may recommend imaging follow-up. If the lesion persists but does not appear to meet the criteria for normal asymmetry, biopsy is warranted. **Invasive lobular carcinoma (ILC)** is notorious for manifesting as subtle asymmetry and is commonly vague and difficult to diagnose.

If your initial mammogram was a 2-D study, additional 3-D imaging is usually very helpful in the workup for asymmetry. If your initial screening mammogram was 3-D, then only ultrasound evaluation may be required at this time because the amount of mammographic information needed to make an assessment has already been acquired on the 3-D study. **Tomosynthesis** (3-D mammography) is particularly useful in this setting.

Breast MRI has become more widely available and may be used to further assess a questionable finding on a standard workup. If biopsy of a lesion is needed, the method of biopsy will be determined by the examination in which the lesion is best seen and by which method is the easiest to perform.

"IS THIS YOU?" SAMPLE CASE SCENARIO

A 36-year-old woman presents for her second **screening mammogram.** She is currently without breast symptoms. She started screening mammograms at age 35 because her mother was diagnosed with breast cancer at age 45 and her maternal grandmother at age 50; therefore, she appropriately initiated screening before age 40.

The patient has a patchy parenchymal pattern that seems more prominent in the **axillary tail** region of the left breast; therefore, she is recalled for additional views. Her examination is reported as **Category 0: Incomplete Evaluation—Additional Imaging Needed**.

She returns the following week for a **diagnostic left mammogram** and directed **left breast ultrasound.**

The **diagnostic mammogram** consists of a full true lateral (90-degree) view, spot compression images in the left MLO view, and rolled CC views. On the additional images the area of previous concern has not persisted as a suspicious abnormality and now has the appearance of normal glandular parenchyma.

Directed **ultrasound** in the area reveals no abnormalities, only normal dense breast parenchyma.

The imaging evaluation is complete and is determined to be **Category 2: Benign.** The patient can return to annual imaging.

Unrelated to her callback but because of her strong family history, this patient would also likely benefit from screening breast MRI. She agrees to discuss this option with her referring physician.

RADIOLOGY CONSULT

A developing or asymmetric density is a common finding on mammography. It may result from overlapping tissue or structures, or it may represent a real lesion (tumor). The purpose of the diagnostic evaluation is to differentiate between the two. Looking at the area from various directions, performing direct compression over the area, and rolling the tissues can help the radiologist determine whether an area represents an overlap or a real lesion. This process may take some doing, but is well worth the time and effort and adds valuable information for the radiologist's interpretation. Tomosynthesis is quite useful in this setting.

F. Architectural Distortion

The normal pattern of the planes and contours of the breast tissue architecture are smooth, undulating, and flowing like waves in the ocean. Distortion is an alteration of that pattern characterized by radiating straight lines from a central point (Fig. 10.8). **Architectural distortion** is commonly seen after surgery of the breast including **excisional biopsy**, **lumpectomy**, **axillary** dissection, and **reduction**, **implant**, and **lift** surgeries. For this reason, technologists are asked to inquire about prior surgeries and to mark any visible scars on the skin so that the interpreting radiologist can correlate the distortion on the film with the history and scar location on the skin.

Distortion can also be seen in an entity called *radial scar*. A radial scar is a benign inflammatory process that causes a focal area of scarring. It is idiopathic (meaning that the cause is not known) but is not the result of surgery. It is sometimes seen in association with breast cancer and may be the only imaging manifestation alerting the radiologist to the abnormality. Often, the tumor itself is not seen but its presence is implied by the distortion.

Sometimes, distortion is suspected but turns out to merely represent overlapping of Cooper's ligaments (connective tissue in the breast that helps maintain its structural integrity) and vessels over areas of normal tissue, giving the impression of criss-crossing lines. Distortion can be difficult to perceive, and practice and experience are required to detect it. It is especially difficult to detect in dense tissue or on a mammogram showing a complex parenchymal pattern (i.e., multiple findings in a random distribution). In my experience, 3-D tomosynthesis significantly improves the radiologist's ability to detect even subtle distortion, improving the ability to find more and even smaller cancers. This is one of the reasons cancer detection increases with the use of 3-D imaging.

The work-up to assess for possible architectural distortion starts with spot compression views to determine whether the area can be effaced or pressed out. Additionally, images in

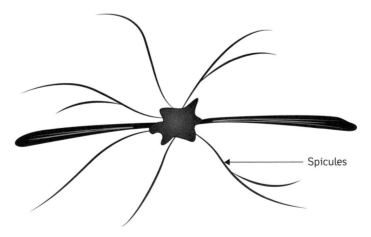

Spicules

FIGURE 10.8 Architectural distortion.

different projections give a better overall view of the area of concern: A true lesion is most likely to be visualized from various angles, whereas overlapping tissue is one-dimensional and is most likely to be seen in only one projection. Although this maxim is not absolute, it is a good general principle to use, with the caveat that occasionally real cancers can be seen in only one plane or projection, so every case should be evaluated with recommendations based on its own merits.

The additional mammographic views may include a true lateral (90-degree) image, angled images at various degrees, rolled views, and so on. If the lesion does not persist in these images, no further workup is needed (i.e., the imaging finding is no longer suspicious). If it persists or if the radiologist wants to verify with another study that the lesion is not an occult (hidden) mass, then ultrasound directed to the area is indicated. The final recommendation can usually be given based on these findings, especially if tomographic imaging is used in the work-up. Breast MRI is occasionally used to clarify findings of possible distortion if the standard imaging is inconclusive or vague.

"IS THIS YOU?" SAMPLE CASE SCENARIO

A 61-year-old woman presents for her annual **screening mammogram**. She denies a history of previous breast surgeries. She is currently without breast symptoms.

She has had previous mammograms, but the films were performed in another state and she does not recall the name of the facility, so no prior films are available for comparison.

An area of distortion is noted in the right breast, and further evaluation of the area is needed. Her examination is reported as **Category 0: Incomplete Evaluation— Additional Imaging Needed**.

The patient is contacted and scheduled for a **diagnostic right mammogram** and possible **right breast ultrasound**. She presents for those evaluations 2 days later.

Additional mammographic views of the right breast are obtained, including a true lateral image and spot compression views in the CC and MLO projections. The area of distortion is vague but persists. The finding is best seen on the tomographic images.

Sonography of the area reveals no discrete or suspicious findings to correlate with the area of concern.

Because of the persistent distortion noted on the mammogram, biopsy is recommended for tissue diagnosis. The evaluation is reported as **Category 4: Suspicious**, and biopsy is recommended. The patient is scheduled for a **stereotactically guided biopsy**.

The patient presents for her **stereotactic biopsy** a week later. She brings to the appointment her prior films performed 3 and 5 years ago, which she found at home in her closet. The films are reviewed by the radiologist, who notes that the distortion was present on the prior films and a scar marker was present that correlated with the distortion. The patient now recalls that she had a surgical biopsy years ago. On closer inspection, she does have a faint, well-healed scar on the right breast.

A scar marker is placed on the patient's skin, and repeat CC and MLO views are performed. These films confirm that the architectural distortion correlates with the site of the previous biopsy, and comparison with the prior films shows that it has been stable. As a result of the new information, the stereotactic biopsy is cancelled.

The radiologist dictates a report to this effect, and the evaluation is now considered to be **Category 2: Benign**. No further workup is indicated, and the patient is returned to annual imaging.

> RADIOLOGY CONSULT
>
> Architectural distortion is never a normal finding—it may be benign, but it is not normal. The question is whether there is a known cause or logical explanation for the distortion. If not, this finding should always be considered suspicious and should warrant investigation even if it has been stable for years. The most common benign cause of architectural distortion is prior surgery or intervention. If the breast tissue has been cut, the normal undulating lines are broken, and the healing and scarring does not usually approximate the presurgical appearance. The purpose of the fibrotic changes of healing is to make the area strong again, not to make it pretty. As a result, surgical scars and healing from other types of trauma can produce a distorted appearance on imaging. If this history is known, then the abnormality is explained by the history. If there is no history, then this finding in the mind of the radiologist represents cancer until proven otherwise. There is a benign process called radial scar that can manifest mammographically as distortion; however, this finding also requires workup and biopsy to prove the benign etiology. The most worrisome finding that manifests as architectural distortion is breast cancer.

2. YOU ARE SYMPTOMATIC OR HAVE A PHYSICAL FINDING

Symptomatic women are among the most anxious of all diagnostic patients because there is a *recognized* clinical complaint or physical finding (i.e., you are aware that there is a problem). As most women would acknowledge, breast symptoms are pretty common and thus mostly physiologic (i.e., a response to normal functioning of the body). However, there are some trends that may help you determine whether your symptoms are more worrisome. In general, symptoms that fluctuate (come and go, increase and decrease in intensity) or are associated with your menstrual cycle are benign and are induced by hormones (mainly estrogen). I find that women taking HRT also commonly report this menstrual-type fluctuation in breast parenchyma even though they are no longer actually having periods. Symptoms that are bilateral, diffuse, and long-standing (chronic) are also more likely to be benign. On the other hand, symptoms that are increasing in intensity, new, or focal are more concerning and definitely warrant evaluation.

The usual scenario comes about when a woman notices a symptom or lump. She reports these symptoms to her referring physician, who then determines what the most appropriate plan of action should be. In the case of benign-type symptoms, it is appropriate to do clinical follow-up with a careful "watch and wait" plan to allow time to observe the symptom. Does it resolve? Does it have the typical presentation of a physiologic response? If the sign or symptom is concerning, a diagnostic work-up is warranted.

Physical findings are also important and may also be recognized on SBE or CBE. A finding or concern first noticed by you is just as important, if not more important, as one by found by your doctor because you have the advantage of being able to examine the area more frequently. I find that women who regularly practice SBE may be able to detect very subtle new changes that are not easily recognizable to others. However, it is the responsibility of the referring physician (a trained professional) to perform an adequate CBE to screen the breast for abnormalities and to evaluate any specific areas of concern brought up by the patient (see Chapter 3). Whether recognized by you or by your doctor, the concerns should be addressed, and a diagnostic evaluation should be performed if those concerns meet certain criteria (see Chapter 8 and Table 8.1).

Special mention should be given to the topic of **fibrocystic disease** or **fibrocystic changes**, which is one of the most confusing conditions for patients, referring doctors, and radiologists. The work-up is widely variable and depends on the overall approach to this entity adopted by the referring physician and the protocols established by the radiologist at the facility in which the imaging evaluation is performed. In my experience, the term *fibrocystic disease* is used incorrectly by many primary care physicians to describe a diffuse and nodular "feel" to the breast on CBE. Having examined literally thousands of breasts, I find that this usually represents the normal, undulating pattern of breast tissue.

I have examined many women who have true fibrocystic breasts, but they are not the majority. I also have seen thousands of mammograms and ultrasound studies and have been able to correlate these imaging patterns with the results of physical examination. This is why performing my own ultrasound studies is so useful. I have the ability to perform an "enhanced" physical examination. The overwhelming majority of women who present with presumed fibrocystic disease in reality have a normal undulating pattern of tissue; what the physician perceives as fibrocystic is in reality Cooper's ligaments, patchy parenchyma, or dense normal tissue. Some women do have true fibrocystic changes that may be evident on mammography, ultrasound, and MRI, but this represents a lower percentage of those presenting with that diagnosis. For this reason, if a woman presents with a diagnosis of "fibrocystic disease" and has no new or focal symptoms, she is treated as a screening patient unless her referring physician believes that a diagnostic evaluation is still warranted. However, if there is a particular area or new area of concern, the workup is, of course, performed with the same diligence as would be used for any other symptomatic patient.

In this section of the chapter, you will be introduced to the common symptoms that might prompt you to come to a breast center for evaluation. These symptoms are pain and swelling, nipple discharge, skin changes, change in breast size, and palpable abnormalities such as a lump or lumpiness, a mass, or thickening. The evaluations for all of these entities are similar and follow the general premise that the evaluation must provide overall screening of the breasts for breast cancer as well as specifically addressing the symptom that prompted the diagnostic evaluation. In most cases, this is accomplished by bilateral mammography (tomosynthesis is very useful in this setting) with additional views of the area of concern, if needed, and ultrasound directed to the area if indicated.

A. Palpable Abnormality (Lump, Mass or Thickening)

Palpable abnormalities should always be subjected to the scrutiny of a diagnostic evaluation unless the finding is stable and has been previously evaluated and found to be benign (e.g., a cyst). It is impossible to determine by physical examination whether a lesion is a cyst or a solid mass—no matter what your doctor says. Although it is true that, along with the patient's age, physical findings such as smooth border, oval or round shape, and easy mobility (meaning that the lesion is easily moved about and is not fixed) do suggest a benign rather than a more suspicious etiology, this is merely an estimate based solely on statistical analysis. I again repeat, it is impossible to discriminate between cystic and solid lesions by physical examination alone. An imaging evaluation is necessary. This situation requires ultrasound confirmation.

A work-up for a palpable abnormality (lump, mass, or thickening) should start with mammography to screen for breast cancer in general and to specifically evaluate the area of concern. If known, the area should be marked with a metallic BB so that the Radiologist can correlate any imaging findings directly with the area of palpable concern (Fig. 10.9). Specific additional views should be added to optimize the visualization of the area, including compression views and sometimes magnification views if calcifications are evident. Directed ultrasound is absolutely needed in this situation if the mammogram shows an abnormality but even more so if there is not a correlative finding on mammography. It is necessary to perform ultrasound in this setting because ultrasound can frequently identify a lesion that is not evident mammographically. If the lesion is believed to be highly concerning for malignancy, surveillance of the rest of the breast is warranted as well as sonographic evaluation of the **axilla** to evaluate the lymph nodes under the arm.

"IS THIS YOU?" SAMPLE CASE SCENARIO

A 26-year-old woman presents with a 3-month history of a fluctuating nodule in the right breast at the 12 **o'clock position**. It is quite tender and is worse just before her cycle. She has no family history of breast or ovarian cancer.

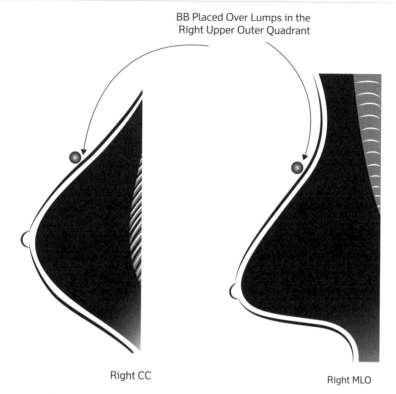

FIGURE 10.9 BB placed on a palpable lump for mammography.

Because of the patient's age and the lack of a concerning family history, her evaluation consists of **ultrasound** only.

Ultrasound reveals a 1.8 cm, homogeneous, well-defined mass along the 12 o'clock axis of the right breast corresponding to the area of concern identified by the patient. Incidental note is made of a similar but smaller, nonpalpable lesion just adjacent to the clinically palpable lesion.

Given the patient's age, no family history, and the imaging findings, the lesions are most likely benign fibroadenomas (the most common benign breast tumor). However, because the larger lesion is palpable, the patient should receive a surgical consultation for discussion of follow-up, needle biopsy, and excisional biopsy options.

Based on the imaging results, the lesion is considered **Category 3: Probably Benign**, and 6- month follow-up would be acceptable. However, because the lesion is palpable, considerations of ultrasound-guided core biopsy or even excision may be warranted based on severity of symptoms or other clinical considerations.

RADIOLOGY CONSULT

If you present for evaluation of a palpable abnormality, consideration should be given to clinical follow-up (i.e., the referring physician examines you repeatedly over a certain period) or surgical consultation, whichever is considered most appropriate by your referring physician. Some referring physicians are comfortable following the physical findings; others are not comfortable with that choice and send all of these women for surgical consultation. Regardless of which method is chosen, palpable abnormalities (if suspicious) should not be ignored, even in the context of benign imaging (i.e., negative mammogram and ultrasound findings), because there are a few types of breast cancer that can manifest as a palpable abnormality with negative imaging—notably, ILC (see Topics in Breast Imaging: Terms About Cancer). Breast MRI has been very helpful in these clinical situations in determining whether a palpable lesion is real. I would use MRI if the lesion is clinically concerning but the standard evaluations with mammography and ultrasound are negative. In this instance, MRI would likely detect a tumor if one is present.

B. Pain and Swelling

Pain is probably the most common breast complaint of women who present for diagnostic evaluation. Although pain is a common symptom (and usually occurs secondary to a benign process), certain types of pain—specifically focal or new pain—should warrant diagnostic evaluation. The rationale for this distinction is that focal pain, although not the typical presentation, may be the presenting symptom that indicates the presence of a cancerous tumor (i.e., when a lesion that is not palpable causes pain in that area of the breast and leads the patient to seek consultation).

Other types of pain may also warrant diagnostic evaluation depending on the patient's or the referring physician's level of concern. Following the general guidelines stated in the first paragraph of this section can help you and your referring physician to better understand the level of concern for the pain. For example, bilateral, fluctuating pain that is associated with menses is less concerning, but focal, new, or intense pain should initiate a diagnostic assessment.

Focal swelling is similar in its presentation and relevance as a palpable lump and should be approached in a similar manner. The workup should proceed as for the evaluation of a palpable abnormality.

"IS THIS YOU?" SAMPLE CASE SCENARIO

A 51-year-old perimenopausal woman presents to the breast center because of increasing focal pain along the 3 o'clock axis of the left breast. The pain has been progressively increasing over the past 2 months. She has a history of fibrocystic changes and has had aspirations in the past. She is not on HRT and is without palpable abnormalities.

The patient sees her gynecologist and is given an order for a **diagnostic bilateral mammogram** and **left breast ultrasound**.

She presents for that evaluation later the same afternoon. **Mammography** reveals that the breast parenchyma is dense bilaterally; however, in the area of concern in the left breast, where a BB marker has been placed (see Fig. 10.9), there are partially obscured nodules. There are no associated calcifications or distortion. The right breast is normal.

Ultrasound of the left breast is performed in the area of concern. Three adjacent simple cysts are seen, corresponding to the area of palpable concern identified by the patient as well as the area of mammographic concern. The dominant cyst measures 2.2 cm.

The imaging evaluation is reported as **Category 2: Benign**. However, because of the patient 's pain—which is focal and severe—**ultrasound-guided cyst aspiration** is performed for symptomatic relief. The patient reports immediate relief of tenderness after aspiration.

She requires no further follow-up and should return to annual imaging.

RADIOLOGY CONSULT

The perimenopausal period can be a bear, to say the least! This is the stage between having regular periods (your ovaries know the routine) and being truly postmenopausal (your ovaries are not producing any more estrogen). This does not happen overnight and can even last for years. What I have found after many years of examining perimenopausal women with imaging is that, if you are prone to fibrocystic changes or have a past history of cysts, frequently there is an exacerbation of these symptoms during this time. My theory is that because the estrogen levels are erratic (up one day, down the next, with no clear pattern), the breasts are hormonally "confused"; this usually resulting in pain and often in an increase in your fibrocystic changes. The good news is that once you are truly postmenopausal, this situation will improve or resolve. All bets are off, though, if you start HRT.

C. Nipple Discharge

Blood coming out of your nipple is, to say the least, one of the most unnerving symptoms that a woman can encounter. This symptom gets women in to see the doctor—fast! What is encouraging is that this symptom is rarely the result of a malignancy, although it does mandate a detailed evaluation because it usually requires surgical biopsy. In past years, women were told to compress their nipples as part of the routine of SBE. What was found was that nipple discharge is common and can be easily expressed by a high percentage of women, especially under conditions of estrogen stimulation (i.e., premenopausal or postmenopausal status on HRT).

Estrogen, which is produced by your ovaries, stimulates fluid production within the breast ducts. When the breast is milked or the nipple is compressed, fluid can be expressed from one or many of the 15 to 20 milk ducts at the tip of the nipple. If you think about this, it makes perfect sense. Evolutionarily, the whole purpose of the breast is to produce fluid milk to feed babies. This is made possible by the production of estrogen, which stimulates the production of milk that can then flow from the nipples—resulting in happy, well-fed babies. When this happens in the context of breastfeeding, it is called *let down* and is seen as normal. It can, however, occur months or years after breastfeeding in some women because the ducts remain patulous (large) and continue to easily discharge or leak fluid. If this occurs from both breasts and from multiple ducts (similar to breastfeeding) but not during the time of lactation, it is usually referred to as *galactorrhea*. It may occur as the result of a pituitary (brain) tumor that produces prolactin, which can be diagnosed with a blood draw and laboratory test or with a brain MRI.

I find that most women report as "discharge" any material that comes from the nipple and is not associated with lactation. Not uncommonly, a pasty, whitish material that can be seen at the tip of a nipple orifice (hole). This is physiologic and is of no clinical significance. The term *discharge* technically refers to liquid that comes out (discharges) from a duct.

Discharge can be either spontaneous (i.e., coming by itself) or nonspontaneous (coming with manual compression). It can be solitary (coming from one duct) or multiductal (coming from many ducts). It can be unilateral (from one breast) or bilateral (from both breasts). And it can be bloody (red) or serous ("like water") or any other color (e.g., brown, yellow, white, green). The most benign and physiologic type of discharge is nonspontaneous, bilateral, multiductal, and not bloody in color. The nature and characteristics of this type of discharge indicate that it is benign by history and is not concerning. The recommendation, then, is "Don't squeeze!" Leave it alone. I cringe sometimes at the maneuvers and the amount of twisting and force some woman use to express this discharge in an effort to demonstrate their "abnormality." In such cases, the discharge may actually be secondary to the trauma that is being inflicted by the woman herself.

At the other end of the spectrum is spontaneous, unilateral, single-duct, bloody discharge. Although this is the scenario that requires the most scrutiny, the results are still overwhelmingly benign. A bloody discharge may be the result of a tumor (papilloma) that grows within the ducts and irritates the lining, causing the duct to bleed. Papillomas are common and benign, but because there is also an entity called *papillary cancer*, all intraductal lesions should be surgically excised. Because most papillary tumors that cause discharge are located within the first 2 cm of the nipple orifice, the standard diagnosis and treatment used to be blind surgical excision (i.e., without imaging guidance) of the first 2 cm of tissue behind the nipple. With better and more advanced studies available to assist in the workup, radiologists can now be more specific and identify the abnormal ductal system before surgery so that it can be specifically targeted. This improves surgical accuracy and decreases excision of unaffected normal tissue.

The imaging work-up for discharge includes the standard mammographic images to screen and assess for breast cancer (which may present as pleomorphic calcifications behind the nipple) as well as directed ultrasound of the nipple and retroareolar area to look for intraductal nodules (i.e., tumors within a milk duct) (Figs. 10.10 and 10.11). If the discharge can be reproduced (i.e., the radiologist is able to squeeze and visually identify the duct location), ductography may performed to see the inside of the duct. Contrast dye is injected into the nipple orifice, which causes the duct containing the dye to appear as a white tube on a subsequent mammogram. A tumor within the duct shows as a defect because the white contrast material surrounds its borders. This is helpful because the location of the discharge does not predict the path of the duct within the breast. For example, a discharge may be coming from the 3 o'clock position of the nipple, but the ductal system within the breast may extend into the 12 o'clock region of the breast.

More recently, breast MRI has been more useful in establishing the presence or absence of disease in the setting of discharge. Sometimes the mammogram and ultrasound findings are completely normal but the MRI result is markedly abnormal. If the symptom profile is concerning and the standard imaging is unremarkable, I very often recommend breast MRI to complete the evaluation. In the setting of suspicious clinical symptoms, a surgical consultation is also warranted because the management of this process, as stated earlier, usually requires surgical management to stop the symptom of discharge and to completely excise the lesion for biopsy.

The workup for discharge should include the following:

Mammography, to screen for breast cancer (specifically, DCIS in the retroareolar region)
Directed ultrasound, to detect intraductal tumors
Ductography, if possible
Breast MRI, as needed based on the clinical concern

Discharge characteristics may be classified as follows:

Benign or physiologic (normal body process)
    Nonspontaneous (requires compression)
    Bilateral (both breasts)
    Multiductal (many holes)
    White, green, brown, or yellow (not bloody)
Concerning
    Spontaneous (comes by itself)
    Unilateral (one breast)
    Single duct (one hole)
    Bloody (red) or serous (clear like water)

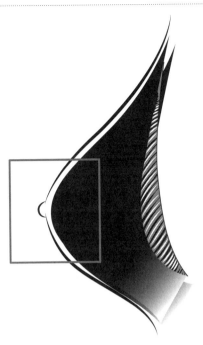

Right ML (true 90° lateral)

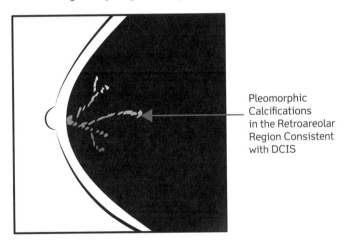

Pleomorphic
Calcifications
in the Retroareolar
Region Consistent
with DCIS

FIGURE 10.10 Mammogram of retroareolar region (history of bloody discharge).

"IS THIS YOU?" SAMPLE CASE SCENARIO

A 37-year-old woman presents with a 2-week history of spontaneous, dark discharge from the right nipple. She is not lactating or pregnant. She denies trauma or mastitis-type symptoms. She has no palpable abnormalities, and a CBE performed by her doctor was also negative. The nipple areolar complex is normal based on visual inspection. Her doctor performed a Hemoccult test which confirmed that the discharging fluid was blood.

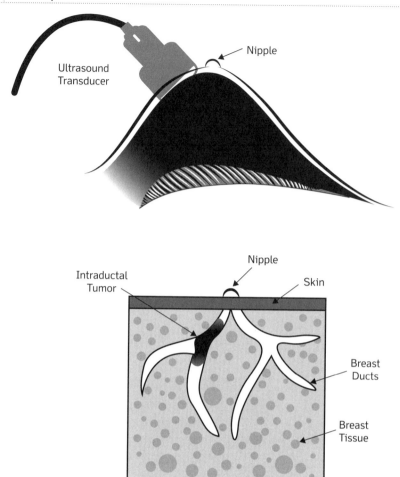

FIGURE 10.11 Ultrasound imaging of intraductal lesion.

A Papanicolaou slide was made of the fluid at the same time, and the results are pending at the time of the imaging evaluation.

Because the patient is older than 30 years of age, she receives a **bilateral diagnostic mammogram** that includes CC, MLO and true lateral open magnification views of the right retroareolar area of the right breast. The true lateral image is performed because papillomas, which are the most common cause of bloody nipple discharge, can appear mammographically as calcifications. Almost all suspicious calcifications require true lateral imaging to exclude milk of calcium as an etiology. In addition, the symptoms could be the result of Paget's disease (in situ cancer within the nipple ducts), and this also would likely manifest mammographically as calcifications, again necessitating a lateral image to complete the assessment (see Fig. 10.10).

The **mammogram** is unremarkable except for an obviously benign nodule in the opposite breast. There are no suspicious findings in the retroareolar area of the right breast that might account for the patient's symptom.

Directed **ultrasound** of the right retroareolar area is unremarkable, and no discrete or solid masses are identified within the ducts.

The patient returns after 2 days and receives a right **ductogram,** which reveals two filling defects within a dilated duct along the 12 o'clock axis.

The imaging evaluation is reported as **Category 4: Suspicious**. Surgical consultation is recommended.

The patient subsequently undergoes **surgical excision** of the area, with the final pathology result confirming benign papilloma. Her discharge resolves after surgery.

RADIOLOGY CONSULT

The diagnostic workup for discharge can vary depending on the clinical symptoms, the patient's age, and the preferences of the surgeon. However, I believe that diagnostic mammography is warranted in almost all cases to exclude obvious malignant-appearing calcifications (in situ cancer) as the cause of the discharge. Also, if the patient may eventually have ductography, she needs to have a full diagnostic mammogram first to serve as a reference. Additionally, ultrasound may reveal intraductal lesions that are not evident mammographically, thus providing a method of image-guided biopsy or localization before surgery. Ductography is quite useful for identifying the location and distribution of the ductal system in question and can provide guidance for localization during surgery (using contrast dye mixed with blue dye). Breast MRI can be valuable for detecting disease that is not evident by other imaging modalities; many times it reveals conditions to be more extensive than initially suggested on standard imaging.

D. Skin Changes

Changes in the skin of the breast may result from either primary breast conditions or primary dermatologic conditions that just happen to affect the skin of the breast. Although there is some overlap in the imaging appearance, there are useful distinctions that may differentiate the two.

Findings that are worrisome and indicative of an underlying breast tumor are **dimpling, retraction, and nipple inversion**. All of these changes, if new or not explained by a previous biopsy, should be considered highly suspicious until proven otherwise. The reasoning is that a cancerous tumor is invading the surrounding tissue and causing a reaction that results in pulling of the skin toward the lesion. This pulling manifests clinically as dimpling, retraction, or inversion. Other changes that are worrisome include wound development on the nipple itself. There is a special type of cancer called Paget's disease that is the result of malignancy in the ducts and immediately around the nipple. This may manifest clinically as a scabbing or wound development on the nipple.

On the other hand, although this is not absolute, skin changes in the areola (the pink or brown pigmented area surrounding the nipple) are usually dermatologic in etiology—caused by psoriasis, eczema, and so on.

Superficial nodules (close to the surface) that are proven to be within the skin are usually diagnosed as sebaceous or inclusion cysts (similar to a pimple). Lesions that are confirmed within the skin are always benign unless the patient has a known malignancy then subcutaneous metastasis should be considered (i.e., cancer from another source that travels to the skin via blood vessels and forms a mass of tumor). Part of the goal of the diagnostic evaluation is to determine the location of a superficial lesion. Is it in the skin and therefore benign, or is it in the superficial portion of the breast tissue (i.e., a breast tissue lesion)? This distinction significantly changes the level of concern and recommendations.

Inflammatory changes in the skin can manifest as thickening of the skin, resulting in an "orange peel" appearance with erythema (redness) and increased warmth. These conditions are discussed in Chapter 11.

"IS THIS YOU?" SAMPLE CASE SCENARIO

A 23-year-old woman presents with a new, superficial, raised area along the 7 o'clock axis of her left breast that was discovered by SBE. She denies insect bites or trauma. She also denies a family history of breast or ovarian cancer.

Given the patient's age, the workup consists of a directed **ultrasound** of the area of concern. Sonography reveals a 5-mm, hypoechoic, oval lesion in the skin of the breast correlating with the area of concern reported by the patient. No underlying parenchymal (breast tissue) abnormalities are noted.

Visual inspection reveals no signs of inflammation or infection.

The area of concern is confirmed to lie within the skin and is consistent with a sebaceous or inclusion cyst. There are no findings to suggest breast malignancy. The evaluation is **Category 2: Benign,** and the patient can commence annual imaging at age 40 unless signs or symptoms prompt earlier reevaluation.

RADIOLOGY CONSULT

Breast ultrasound is a must when one is trying to determine whether a superficial lesion is actually in the skin or in the breast tissue near the skin. Many times, this distinction is difficult to determine by physical examination alone. However, the determination is critical because, except for rare circumstances of subcutaneous metastais, skin lesions are benign and are not at all concerning for breast cancer. With these lesions, although dermatology consultation may be required, biopsy to exclude breast cancer is not needed—the location has essentially excluded that as an etiology. On the other hand, a lesion in the superficial tissues of the breast is a breast tumor that, like all breast tumors, must be evaluated to determine its level of suspicion for breast cancer. The level of suspicion may be none (it is a cyst), low (it is a fibroadenoma), or suspicious (it is a cancer). If it is unclear whether the lesion is in the skin or in the parenchymal tissues of the breast, biopsy may be needed for tissue diagnosis.

E. Change in Breast Size

Weight changes and hormone status changes can certainly affect the size of the breasts, for better or for worse! However, these overall systemic changes affect the breasts symmetrically (i.e., both breasts are affected equally). What is abnormal is to have one breast change relative to its normal size or in comparison with the other breast. Either increased or decreased size of one breast relative to the other is concerning and should be investigated.

One of the sneakiest types of breast cancer, ILC, can manifest as a subtle, overall decrease in the size of the breast—called the *shrinking breast*. This cancer can infiltrate large portions of the breast before it is noticed clinically by you, by your doctor, or by imaging; the findings may be quite subtle until the cancer is widespread. You are actually the best monitor of this type of symptom because you have access to inspect your breasts on a regular basis. Another bad actor is inflammatory breast cancer that is by definition stage 4 disease (the latest stage, with the poorest prognosis); it may manifest identically to mastitis, causing overall enlargement of the breast secondary to the inflammatory component and the extensive tumor load in the breast itself.

"IS THIS YOU?" SAMPLE CASE SCENARIO

A 52-year-old woman presents for **MRI** evaluation due to shrinking size of her left breast.

The patient's history is significant in that she had a diagnosis of invasive lobular cancer of the left breast at age 50 but declined conventional therapy (i.e., surgery, chemotherapy, and radiation therapy). She consulted a naturopathic doctor and opted for natural treatment with an emphasis on diet, supplements, and injections. She states that the tumor, which at that time was 2 cm in diameter, resolved with this treatment, and she was in her usual state of being until 3 months ago, when she noticed that her left breast was firm and smaller in size compared to the right.

The usual workup would entail **mammography** and **ultrasound,** but the patient declines, citing her concerns about the risks of radiation associated with mammography.

She states that she will allow only one imaging study. In order to get the most "bang for the buck" in evaluating the extensive disease in the affected breast and associated skin, axillary lymph node, and chest wall involvement, it was decided that **breast MRI** would best serve the needs of the patient and provide the most information for her surgeon and oncologist.

Not surprisingly, the **MRI** reveals extensive, irregular and nodular, washout-type enhancement within all quadrants of the breast. The tumor extends to the pectoralis muscle (chest wall) and into the cleavage region. Skin enhancement is most prominent within the anterior aspect of the breast but is also extensive and extends into the axillary region and the cleavage area. Matted, enlarged, enhancing lymph nodes are also observed.

Given the extent of disease, the patient is not a candidate for immediate surgery, and soon after the examination she starts neoadjuvant chemotherapy (i.e., chemotherapy given before surgery).

The **MRI** also shows an incidental solid mass in the liver, and **contrast-enhanced computed tomography (CT) is** recommended to assess for possible liver metastasis.

RADIOLOGY CONSULT

Unilateral change in breast size should always prompt an assessment, even if the patient is the only one who notices. Certainly, benign inflammation such as mastitis can cause a change in breast size, but this also should be evaluated and confirmed to have resolved completely before the issue can be put to rest. I also sometimes see patients whose normal asymmetry of breast size becomes more noticeable after they gain or lose a significant amount of weight. Of course, gathering an accurate clinical history, performing a thorough physical evaluation, completing the appropriate imaging evaluation, and providing close clinical follow-up are key to differentiating benign etiologies from more sinister ones. For instance, if the findings on standard imaging (mammography and ultrasound) are benign but there is persistent clinical concern, breast MRI can be helpful. If MRI reveals an obvious abnormality, the patient will undergo a biopsy and there will be no delay in diagnosis. A negative MRI result will add support for clinical follow-up if the clinical suspicion is low, thus lessening the patient's anxiety and supporting the referring physician's decision to follow the patient.

3. YOU HAVE A HISTORY THAT REQUIRES SPECIAL ATTENTION

Sometimes a patient's prior history necessitates a diagnostic evaluation even if there are no new or current breast symptoms. The history itself is sufficient to determine that special attention needs to be afforded to the examination because of a specific issue or established protocol. These situations are described in the following paragraphs.

A. Surveillance of a Previous Lesion Reported as Probably Benign

Imaging surveillance (i.e., serial images obtained at certain intervals over a determined time frame) is a practice that is one of the best researched approaches in breast imaging. If this practice is followed based on established guidelines, it can serve as a legitimate alternative to biopsy with no harm to you, the patient. It does, however, require an understanding of the concept by you and your referring doctor to limit the anxiety associated with not having an immediate definitive answer (i.e., from biopsy) and the anticipation associated with the follow-up examinations. This allows you a sense of peace between examinations (i.e., feeling that you are not harming yourself and that you are making a reasonable choice).

"Probably benign" does not mean, "I don't know." It means that the radiologist has performed a thorough evaluation, reviewed your films, and reported a finding that is very likely not cancer but does not have the features that are "characteristically" benign. If certain criteria are followed, the statistical likelihood of cancer is less than 2%. In other words, more than 98% of the lesions designated as "probably benign" and placed in surveillance will turn out to be truly benign. If, during the surveillance period, there is a change in the lesion (usually increasing size or development of a less well-defined contour), a biopsy will be recommended. The less than 2% of lesions that are subsequently proven to be malignant will still be in an early stage (stage 0 or stage 1) and thus likely curable with no harm done. (Stage refers to how far the disease has progressed; it is not changed or affected by "delay" in diagnosis.)

I find that once this strategy is explained to patients, they are much more appreciative of the fact that the goal is to be accurate but to defer biopsy (which does have some associated minor risks) if it is not needed. Although we could biopsy all lesions that are visible or targetable, it is imperative to use discretion when recommending biopsy. As **percutaneous** biopsies have become perfected and complications have lessened, many patients and doctors seem less likely to tolerate any uncertainty—sometimes to the detriment of the patient, as when needle biopsy leads to a bleeding complication or infection, however rare. I have even encountered some referring doctors who do not "believe" in surveillance and vigorously counsel their patients against it because of their lack of understanding of the rationale and supporting literature.

The criteria established by for "Probably Benign" lesions are as follows:

Nonpalpable focal asymmetry with concave margins and interspersed fat
Nonpalpable, solid, oval or round, predominantly well-defined nodule
Round or oval calcifications
Multiple (>3) similar findings, which may be bilateral

If, after a full diagnostic evaluation based on the standard of care for your age and clinical situation, the lesion is believed to be "probably benign," a short-interval follow-up will be recommended. The literature supports a 6-month follow-up interval. This has two advantages. First, it allows enough time so that if there is a change from the initial study, it will be obvious enough to be perceived visually by the radiologist. Second, 6 months is a relatively short period of time in the natural history of a breast cancer, so even if the lesion is subsequently proven to be malignant, your prognosis will be the same. After the

6-month examination, you will return to the annual protocol, and the area of concern will be specifically addressed for a total of 2 years. Two years of stability in essence establishes the benign nature of the lesion without the need for biopsy.

"IS THIS YOU?" SAMPLE CASE SCENARIO

A 40-year-old woman has a baseline **bilateral screening mammogram** in January 2014. An oval nodule is noted in the right breast.

She is recalled for **diagnostic mammography** and **ultrasound**, which reveal favorable characteristics.

The lesion is characterized as **Category 3: Probably Benign**, and a 6-month follow-up **mammogram** is recommended.

The patient returns in July 2014, and a **diagnostic unilateral right mammogram** reveals the nodule to be stable.

In January 2015, she presents for annual follow-up imaging, which consists of a **diagnostic bilateral mammogram** with an additional view of the right breast lesion which reveals that the nodule has remained stable.

In January 2016, she is again due for annual surveillance imaging and has a **diagnostic bilateral mammogram** with an additional view of the right breast lesion. The nodule is again found to be stable.

The patient has now completed her surveillance period; the lesion continues to have favorable characteristics and has been stable for 2 years. Her assessment is now reported as **Category 2: Benign,** and she can return to a schedule of annual **screening mammograms.**

RADIOLOGY CONSULT

Breast radiologists try hard to be as definitive a possible: The finding is benign ("see you next year") or the finding is suspicious (needs biopsy). To make this decision, a thorough workup is imperative and may include mammography, ultrasound, or even breast MRI. However, there are times when the probability of malignancy is very low but the lesion is not clearly benign based on characteristics; in such cases, follow-up surveillance (rather than a biopsy) is appropriate. If you and your referring physician understand the reasoning behind the recommendation and realize that is not an "I don't know" category, you can comfortably and calmly accept this recommendation as a well-informed patient.

B. Follow-up of a Previous Benign Biopsy

When a biopsy is performed, either by needle or by surgery, actual tissue is retrieved. After the pathology result becomes available, the performing physician assesses the sampling result as to accuracy (Did I sample the correct lesion?), adequacy (Did I get enough tissue?), and whether the tissue diagnosis is **concordant** with the imaging lesion (Does the pathology diagnosis *explain* the targeted imaging abnormality?). All of this review and correlation should be performed in the immediate postbiopsy period (1-2 weeks). If the lesion is confirmed to be benign, the patient can usually be placed back into a routine screening protocol. Sometimes, however, it is necessary to perform a follow-up study, either to confirm a continued or decreasing benign appearance or to reestablish a new baseline appearance (i.e., if the architecture has been altered by the biopsy).

If follow-up is recommended, the interval is usually 6 months. The follow-up study may be a mammogram, ultrasound, or MRI, depending on the method of biopsy. Some would argue that all percutaneous biopsies require follow-up to look for missed cancers due to inaccurate or inadequate sampling. This is becoming less necessary given the advances in methods and review of biopsy results from the more established percutaneous methods such as stereotactic biopsy and ultrasound biopsy. Newer methods of biopsy, such as MRI, have a less robust literature regarding long-term follow-up, so follow-up after this type of biopsy may be still warranted. Even if the imaging and pathology findings are concordant, it is always at the discretion of the radiologist to request a follow-up study based on experience and familiarity with a certain method of biopsy, nonspecific findings on the pathology report, or the standard protocol established by the breast care facility (Topics in Breast Imaging: Terms About Biopsy Results).

"IS THIS YOU?" SAMPLE CASE SCENARIO

A 53-year-old woman has a successful **stereotactic biopsy** for an RUOQ density in July 2015; the lesion was found on her screening examination a month earlier. The final pathology report reveals benign parenchyma and fibrosis. The imaging and pathology findings are believed to be concordant (i.e., the pathology report explains the imaging finding). The patient had started HRT in January of 2015, and the density, although new, has a mammographic appearance similar to that of glandular tissue. This pathology report therefore confirms the benign nature of this new finding. A **6-month mammographic follow-up** is recommended.

The patient returns in February 2016 (a bit late, because of the holiday bustle) for her follow-up imaging. She is without breast symptoms.

A **diagnostic unilateral right diagnostic mammogram** is performed; it consists of the routine CC and MLO views as well as an MLO spot view of the area of previous biopsy. The previous lesion is now less conspicuous (less evident), and the clip that was placed at the time of the biopsy is seen at the biopsy site. There are no suspicious findings in the remainder of the breast.

The evaluation is reported as **Category 2: Benign**, and the patient is returned to annual imaging. In June 2016, she will be due a bilateral **screening mammogram**.

RADIOLOGY CONSULT

Because of the ongoing experience and long-term study of percutaneous biopsy results and pathology correlation, there are now times when short-interval follow-up may not be necessary if all of the strict criteria for assessing the radiolologic-pathologic correlation are met. This conclusion is somewhat controversial, however. I feel very comfortable in some instances placing a patient who has undergone needle biopsy with benign results back into an annual imaging protocol. That being said, I usually recommend a 6-month follow-up period after biopsy to reestablish the new baseline appearance (and this is the protocol established at our facility). The decision to continue with follow-up is really at the discretion of the performing radiologist and is never a wrong or bad idea in these circumstances. If I have any concern about the correlation, however, I recommend surgical biopsy instead of follow-up. Although medicine is a science, it is also an art, and artists are allowed some individual expression. They also need to be able to sleep at night without regret or worry about missing or delaying a breast cancer diagnosis.

C. History of Breast Cancer, Especially Lumpectomy

If you are a woman who has had a diagnosis of breast cancer, you can legitimately be a "diagnostic" patient now and forever. The surgical treatment of the cancer will determine the type and frequency of imaging needed to manage your particular situation. If you have had breast conservation therapy (i.e., lumpectomy or partial mastectomy), you will definitely require imaging follow-up to assess for recurrence in the treated breast, which by definition has been proven to have a propensity to develop cancer. Because of the statistical probabilities of recurrence at the biopsy site with breast conservation surgery, the surgical site and the involved breast will be given special attention for a certain period thereafter. Findings that may be common after lumpectomy include distortion and deformity or a mass-like cavity at the surgical site. Findings that are commonly seen after radiation include skin thickening and trabecular thickening (thickening of the breast tissue strands) (Fig. 10.12). Although the time frame can vary based on interpretations of the literature and conventions within a specialty, the time interval and protocol should be consistent within a particular facility. All of the radiologists in a facility should be following a similar recommendation protocol that is consistent with others in their practice and with the standards in their local area.

In my practice, we have determined that 5 years is an acceptable time frame in which to do special investigation of the lumpectomy site given that recurrence is most likely during this period. The patient continues annual imaging but additionally receives spot and/or magnification views of the lumpectomy bed (i.e., the site of surgery). This is done to look for subtle changes or findings that might identify a recurrent malignancy. Some referring physicians request follow-up films every 6 months. After 5 years, the patient can return to annual screening, but she or her referring doctor may elect to continue annual imaging

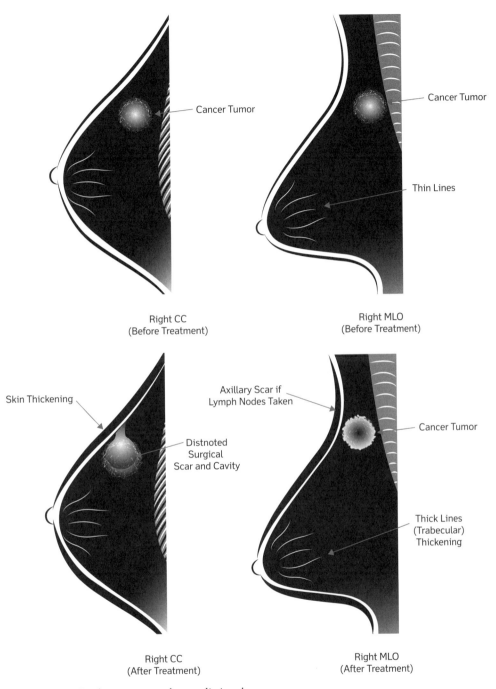

Cancer Tumor

Cancer Tumor

Thin Lines

Right CC
(Before Treatment)

Right MLO
(Before Treatment)

Skin Thickening

Axillary Scar if
Lymph Nodes Taken

Distnoted
Surgical
Scar and Cavity

Cancer Tumor

Thick Lines
(Trabecular)
Thickening

Right CC
(After Treatment)

Right MLO
(After Treatment)

FIGURE 10.12 Postlumpectomy and postradiation changes.

as diagnostic. If so, the examinations will be performed when a radiologist is available to immediately review the films and request additional work-up as needed at the time of the appointment. I personally prefer this method. In my practice, if the evaluation is performed as a diagnostic, I also make ultrasound a part of the annual surveillance after a breast cancer lumpectomy surgery; this provides for both lumpectomy site assessment and a more complete breast screening.

If you have had mastectomy with either no **reconstruction** or reconstruction with implants, you require no mammographic screening. However, some women opt for sonographic screening or MRI screening. If you have had a mastectomy with **TRAM reconstruction**, the literature shows that mammography screening has some benefit. The unaffected breast (**contralateral** side) requires annual screening only.

Referring doctors, especially surgeons and oncologists, usually have established protocols and request for imaging follow-up based on their unique situation or practice; these requests should obviously be honored (also see Chapter 14).

The following guidelines summarize my preferred mammographic follow-up relative to the surgical treatment:

Mastectomy without reconstruction   No mammogram
Mastectomy with implant reconstruction   No mammogram
Mastectomy with TRAM reconstruction   Mammogram
Lumpectomy   Mammogram

"IS THIS YOU?" SAMPLE CASE SCENARIO

A 68-year-old woman is diagnosed with left breast malignancy (high-grade DCIS with focal microinvasion) in January 2016 based on the presence of calcifications noted on a routine **screening mammogram** performed in December 2015. She undergoes lumpectomy in February 2016 and presents to the breast center in April 2016 for imaging evaluation before receiving radiation therapy.

The patient receives a left **diagnostic mammogram** that includes the routine CC and MLO views but also a full lateral view and spot magnification views in the CC and true lateral projections. The spot views are necessary to provide additional, directed evaluation of the lumpectomy bed to better assess for subtle changes at the surgical site. The lumpectomy bed requires special scrutiny because it is an area in the breast that has a proven propensity to make cancers and therefore a statistically higher risk of developing cancer compared with the rest of the breast. The true lateral images are needed for assessment of any potential calcifications because the patient's malignancy was evidenced mammographically as calcifications.

The lumpectomy bed (i.e., cavity, scarring, and associated distortion) is evident mammographically as a new, irregular density with distortion. Four clips are seen within the new finding, and the finding correlates exactly with a scar marker that was placed on the patient's skin by the performing technologist. Both of these results confirm that the new, irregular density with distortion correlates with the patient's surgical bed (lumpectomy site). Therefore, this is an expected postsurgical finding and is not believed to be suspicious.

However, at the lateral margin of the lumpectomy bed, a linearly oriented cluster of pleomorphic calcifications is visualized. They do not layer on the lateral views. These calcifications are believed to be suspicious for malignancy.

The interesting question here is whether these calcifications are residual (i.e., were present previously but were not completely excised at the time of the initial surgery) or new (i.e., representing interval development of cancer within a short time after adequate surgical treatment).

On review of the patient's prior (presurgical) mammograms and the specimen radiograph performed at the time of the surgery, the calcifications on the current mammogram do appear to be new, not residual. Therefore, they represents a rapid, short-interval recurrence. The evaluation is reported as **Category 5: Highly Suspicious**, and **stereotactically guided needle biopsy** is recommended.

A pathology report from the subsequent **stereotactic biopsy** confirms the calcifications to be high-grade DCIS.

Breast MRI is also performed and reveals no other areas of suspicious findings. However, given the diagnosis of recurrent cancer, the patient opts for mastectomy.

RADIOLOGY CONSULT

The survival rate for women with breast cancer who undergo breast conservation therapy (i.e., lumpectomy) is the same as for women who have a mastectomy (i.e., removal of the entire breast). However, in the case of breast conservation therapy, the remaining portion of the breast has to be monitored for evidence of recurrence (i.e., a new cancer in the same breast within a specified time frame) so that prompt treatment can occur. Because recurrence rates are highest within the first 5 years after lumpectomy, radiologists at my institution obtain additional views of the lumpectomy site whenever the patient receives a mammogram during that time interval. If, after 5 years, there has been no evidence of recurrence, the patient is returned to more routine imaging. This usually means a resumption of annual imaging, which may be performed as a diagnostic or a screening study, depending on the preference of the ordering physician. I personally prefer that these patients have diagnostic evaluations for an extended period or indefinitely.

D. Incidental Finding Seen in the Breast on a Non-breast Study

Occasionally, apparent lesions are seen in the breast tissue on radiologic studies performed for assessment of other parts of the body. This occurs most commonly with CT of the chest and whole-body positron emission tomography (PET), both of which image structures near the breasts and therefore may include breast tissue in the image.

CT is used to evaluate the lungs and chest structures. Because of its proximity to the chest wall, breast tissue is usually included in the field of view. The breast tissue is not compressed and can have a mass-like appearance that merely represents uncompressed normal tissue. However, if the appearance is mass like or asymmetric, a workup in the breast center is warranted.

Whole-body PET is a nuclear medicine molecular study that is performed in cancer patients to look for cancer activity in parts of the body other than the primary site (i.e., evidence of metastatic disease). Whole-body PET for thyroid, lung, or other cancers may reveal incidental lesions in the breast tissue. One study by Korn and May revealed that when women presented for a breast imaging evaluation as a result of their PET study, a high percentage (83%) actually had an unsuspected breast cancer diagnosed.

Because neither CT nor PET is an adequate study to appropriately evaluate breast lesions, there should always be a recommendation for a standard evaluation with established breast imaging modalities such as mammography, ultrasound, and/or MRI to determine the level of concern.

"IS THIS YOU?" SAMPLE CASE SCENARIO

A 43-year-old woman who was diagnosed with thyroid cancer 1 year ago presents for a **whole-body PET** scan as a part of her routine follow-up to assess for possible metastatic disease.

Although no thyroid lesions or other findings suspicious for metastatic thyroid cancer are found, intense activity is noted within the left breast. The woman is without breast symptoms. Her last **screening mammogram** was 2 years ago.

She is scheduled for a breast imaging evaluation including a **diagnostic bilateral mammogram** and **left breast ultrasound**.

The **mammogram** reveals a 2-cm, spiculated mass in the LUOQ.

The lesion is confirmed to be a solid, irregular mass by **ultrasound**.

The evaluation is highly suspicious for a primary breast malignancy within the left breast and is reported as **Category 5: Highly Suspicious. Ultrasound-guided core biopsy** is recommended.

Two days later, the patient has the **ultrasound-guided core biopsy**, and the tissue samples are sent to the laboratory for analysis and interpretation by the pathologist.

Three days after that, the pathology report is available and confirms the diagnosis of primary breast malignancy: IDC, grade 2.

The patient is currently without clinical evidence of thyroid cancer.

E. Search for the Primary Tumor in a Patient with Metastatic Disease

Radiologists are occasionally asked to evaluate a woman who has undergone biopsy of another organ, such as the liver, and whose pathology findings have revealed an adenocarcinoma suggestive of metastasis from another organ (i.e., not a primary liver cancer). Adenocarcinomas that commonly originate from the lung, stomach, kidney, breast, and ovary are considerations. Because management and treatment vary depending on the original site of the cancer (primary source), a search begins to determine the primary tumor location. To this end, the patient presents to the breast center with an order stating "Looking for Primary." This requires a bilateral diagnostic breast evaluation, which is performed with the supervision of the radiologist so that any questionable areas can be immediately evaluated and additional mammographic films and ultrasound studies can be performed at the same appointment.

"IS THIS YOU?" SAMPLE CASE SCENARIO

A 63-year-old woman presents to her primary physician with the complaint of abdominal pain concerning for gallbladder disease.

An **abdominal ultrasound** study is performed and reveals gallstones and also multiple, solid-appearing lesions within the liver.

To further characterize the liver lesions, **abdominal CT** with and without contrast enhancement is performed. The liver lesions are variably enhancing and are present in both lobes. The largest is in the posterior aspect of the right lobe.

The patient undergoes **CT-guided needle biopsy** of the right liver lesion, and the pathology findings reveal adenocarcinoma consistent with a metastatic process. In other words, this is not a primary liver cancer but cancer from another source that has traveled to the liver via blood vessels or lymphatics.

The patient is scheduled for a breast evaluation including a **diagnostic bilateral mammogram** and **bilateral breast ultrasound**.

Mammography reveals an area of density and calcifications within the right breast as well as increased size and density of a lower axillary lymph node when compared with the patient's previous mammogram performed 14 months earlier.

Ultrasound reveals an irregular, poorly defined mass corresponding to the mammographic lesion and also an axillary lymph node with a thickened cortex.

The evaluation is concerning for a primary breast malignancy with metastatic infiltration of the axillary lymph node. It is reported as **Category 5: Highly Suspicious**. A two-site **ultrasound-guided core biopsy** is recommended.

The next day, the patient undergoes **ultrasound-guided core biopsy** of both the breast lesion and the axillary lymph node. The tissue samples are sent to the laboratory for analysis and interpretation by the pathologist.

Two days after that, the pathology report is available and confirms the diagnosis of primary breast malignancy (IDC, grade 3) as well as metastatic disease within the lymph node.

RADIOLOGY CONSULT

Although these "search and find" cases could technically be done as screening examinations (i.e., in an asymptomatic patient), I prefer to perform them as diagnostic evaluations. In this situation, a patient with high anxiety (due to her recent diagnosis of cancer) is coming to the breast care facility to "find the source." A callback in this situation would be unsettling for the patient in terms of her state of mind. For this reason, I perform a diagnostic evaluation, review the films immediately, perform any additional studies as needed (including ultrasound), and report the findings (good or bad) to the patient at that time.

11

Breast Urgent-cies

THIS CANNOT WAIT UNTIL TOMORROW!

THERE ARE FEW true emergencies in breast imaging. Some are urgent, and most are important, but they rarely are emergent. Suspected breast abscesses are a clear exception; they warrant immediate attention and sometimes require drainage. These patients usually are seen on the same day for evaluation and treatment. Drainage (i.e., puncturing with a needle and aspirating fluid or pus) is performed for symptom relief, and the material is collected and sent to the laboratory for analysis so that an antibiotic can be tailored to the causative organism.

Other urgent symptoms that warrant immediate attention include inflammation that suggests acute or active mastitis (i.e., breast infection), inflammatory cancer, and significant implant issues such as a postoperative complication or inflammation from an acute rupture. The patient may have a hot, red, swollen, and tender breast. This often is accompanied by constitutional symptoms such as fever, chills, and general malaise or fatigue. The patient may feel as if she is coming down with a cold or the flu. These conditions can make the breasts exceedingly tender and, depending on the situation, may require hospitalization. Immediate medical management may be necessary, including antibiotics and pain medications.

The caveat in this situation is that mastitis, which is common, and inflammatory breast cancer, which is less common but significantly more serious, can have identical symptoms (i.e., red, hot, and tender breast with skin thickening). These patients usually can tolerate only ultrasound evaluation because of the extreme tenderness, but ultrasound assessment is useful to exclude a drainable abscess (i.e., pocket of pus) (Fig. 11.1).

Close watchful waiting is the key to management of these conditions. The required end point is complete (not just improved) resolution of symptoms. I use 2 months as the outside timeframe. If the symptoms do not completely resolve by that time, a biopsy

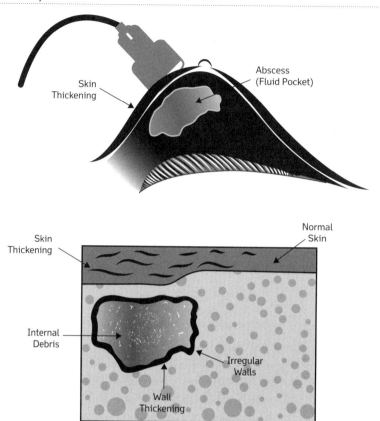

FIGURE 11.1 Breast abscess.

should be performed to exclude inflammatory breast cancer as a cause. This is usually a punch biopsy of the skin performed by the surgeon or a needle biopsy performed by the radiologist if there is an identifiable area to target on ultrasound. If the woman's symptoms do resolve, I prefer to bring the patient back within 2 months for a follow-up examination and to complete the imaging evaluation. By this time, she can tolerate the compression needed for mammography, and the radiologist can determine that there are no mammographic findings suggesting malignancy. Management then proceeds based on her symptoms without concern that she has a cancer mimicking mastitis.

Other same-day evaluations can include elderly or debilitated patients and patients from out of town with a very suspicious finding. For them, returning at a later time would be difficult or could significantly delay the diagnosis of an obvious cancer.

Patients who have undergone recent implant surgery may require immediate evaluation at the breast center to assess postsurgical complications such as an infection or abscess or bleeding around the implant. Ultrasound is a useful and readily available tool for assessing these abnormalities.

Postoperative patients undergoing excisional biopsy, lumpectomy, or mastectomy may require immediate evaluation if operative complications are suspected. Ultrasound is the most useful imaging tool in this setting. Ultrasound guidance can be used for drainage of fluid collections resulting from infection to provide relief from the pressure of fluid buildup. Collected fluid also can be sent to the laboratory to determine the type of infection and thus help direct treatment.

RADIOLOGY CONSULT

One of my concerns about women who have mastitis-type symptoms is that they are referred from a wide range of clinicians with various degrees of knowledge and experience in the management of mastitis or other breast conditions. For some less-experienced providers, clinical improvement in symptoms may be seen as confirmation of a diagnosis of benign mastitis, and close watchful follow-up may not occur because there is no heightened awareness of the less likely but possible diagnosis of inflammatory cancer. I have seen a few patients who improved on antibiotic therapy and had recurrent flares over a period of months to a year or two who were eventually diagnosed with inflammatory breast cancer. They were typically younger patients for whom it was reasonable to assume that benign mastitis was the correct diagnosis. However, complete resolution must be the end point for the referring clinician, even in pregnant and lactating women. Otherwise, referral to a breast surgeon is prudent.

12

You Need a Biopsy—Don't Panic!

IMAGE-GUIDED NEEDLE BIOPSY: A REMARKABLE

ADVANCE IN TECHNOLOGY AND PATIENT CARE

THE DEVELOPMENT OF image-guided needle procedures is one of the most remarkable advances in medicine and particularly in breast imaging. The ability to obtain tissue with minimal risk and complication and in much shorter timeframes has revolutionized the process of tissue acquisition for diagnosis of breast conditions. The guidance methods used for these procedures include **mammography** (i.e., stereotactic method), **ultrasound** (i.e., sonographic method), and breast **magnetic resonance imaging (MRI)**. The type of guidance used is determined by how the lesion is best seen (and most easily targeted) and the ease of performing the biopsy. Ultrasound is the quickest and most efficient method and is used for most needle biopsy procedures.

Before image-guided procedures became the standard of care, most breast lesions required surgical biopsy for diagnosis. In some cases, women had **bilateral** (double) **mastectomies** for benign fibrocystic disease, a condition that we now easily diagnose and treat with minimal intervention.

This chapter explains the basic preparation needed for image-guided biopsies and discusses each type of procedure and the radiologic criteria used to confirm the accuracy of the biopsy, including proof that the lesion sampled was the one targeted. Needle-guided **cyst aspiration** and fluid-drainage procedures also are reviewed.

Lesion Choice

Abnormal imaging findings that require biopsy are by definition suspicious, which can mean mildly suspicious (i.e., it is unlikely to be cancer but cancer must be excluded), moderately suspicious (i.e., **benign** or **malignant** findings are about equally possible), or very suspicious (i.e., it is considered cancer until proven otherwise). Arriving at the final diagnosis has become much easier with the development of image-guided needle biopsy.

With imaging by mammography, ultrasound, or MRI, radiologists can visualize the lesion to target it. They have a way to accurately put a needle into the lesion and retrieve sample material, which is then sent to the laboratory for processing. The **pathologist** (i.e., a doctor trained in the assessment of cells and disease processes) looks at the cells under the microscope, makes an assessment about their makeup, and decides whether they are cancerous or benign.

Ultrasound-Guided Core Biopsy

After reviewing the diagnostic breast images, the radiologist may recommend a breast biopsy to diagnose an area of concern seen on the ultrasound scan. Ultrasound-guided breast biopsy is a minimally invasive, highly accurate method used to obtain small samples of breast tissue for evaluation. Ultrasound (i.e., sonography) does not involve the use of x-rays and allows the radiologist to remove samples quickly and accurately (Fig. 12.1). The tissue is sent to the laboratory for evaluation by a pathologist, and the results usually are available within a few business days. Most breast biopsies (approximately 80%) do not result in a cancer diagnosis, but tissue sampling is required to make an accurate determination.

RISKS AND BENEFITS

This procedure is reliable, less invasive, less costly, and less complicated than surgical biopsy according to the American College of Surgeons. It does not require general

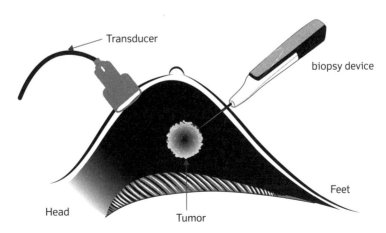

FIGURE 12.1 Ultrasound-guided core biopsy.

anesthesia or stitches, and it can be used to evaluate lumps under the arm or near the chest wall, which can be difficult to access with other methods.

Because a small nick is being made in the skin, there is a slight (less than 1%) risk of bleeding and infection. For women with breast implants, there is a very small risk of implant rupture during the biopsy. As with other types of biopsy, there is a remote possibility that the tissue removed will not provide adequate information for diagnosis, in which case a surgical biopsy will be necessary.

WHAT TO EXPECT

This simple procedure is usually performed in an office setting. The entire process takes slightly more than 1 hour, but the biopsy itself takes only a few minutes. It is advisable to discontinue taking ibuprofen (Advil, Motrin), naproxen (Aleve), aspirin, fish oil, and vitamin E at least 5 to 7 days before the biopsy. If you are taking prescription medications that affect blood clotting (e.g., Coumadin, Plavix), contact your physician to obtain permission to stop these medications for 3 to 5 days before the biopsy to minimize possible bleeding complications.

You should wear comfortable clothing; only the top portion needs to be removed. Wearing a sports-type bra will be helpful after the procedure. Eat a light meal beforehand. You may drive to the appointment. On arrival, you will be asked to change into a gown and to sign a consent form for the biopsy.

During the biopsy, you lie on your back, the area of concern is scanned by the technologist, and the result is shown to the radiologist. The radiologist then cleans and numbs the relevant area of your breast with a local anesthetic to prevent discomfort during the biopsy. As the area is numbed, you will feel a stinging sensation for a few seconds.

A very small incision is made in the skin, and the tissue samples are obtained. In most cases, a small marker or clip is placed in the breast to identify the area of the biopsy. After the biopsy, pressure is applied to the area for a few minutes to stop bleeding. A low-pressure mammogram is done to document placement of the marker because it may be needed for future localization. If the lesion was seen on a mammogram, this post-procedure film can confirm that the targeted lesion was actually biopsied. Steri-Strips (i.e., medical tape) and gauze dressing are used at the end of the procedure to cover the biopsy area.

You will be discharged with an ice pack and written instructions to take home. Acetaminophen (Tylenol) may be used to relieve discomfort. You should avoid lifting or strenuous activity on biopsy day and the next day. Most women resume their normal activities the following day. Some tenderness and bruising are common for the first few days after the biopsy.

(Adapted with Permission from LuAnn Roberson, RN, BSN, CN-BN)

Stereotactically Guided Needle Biopsy

After reviewing the diagnostic breast images, the radiologist may recommend that you have a breast biopsy to diagnose an area of concern that was found on the mammogram. Mammography is the gold standard examination for early detection of breast cancer; it can often detect an abnormality long before it can be felt by you or your health care provider.

Stereotactically guided breast biopsy is a minimally invasive, highly accurate procedure guided by mammography that is used to obtain small samples of breast tissue for evaluation (a simplified rendering is seen in Fig. 12.2). It is most helpful when the mammogram reveals clustered or linear microcalcifications, a new tissue distortion that was not seen on previous mammograms, or a mass that cannot be felt or seen with ultrasound imaging. This type of biopsy uses mammographic images taken from three angles to aid in calculating the exact location of the tissue to be sampled.

The procedure is performed by a radiologist. The tissue sample is sent to the laboratory for evaluation by a pathologist. The results usually are available within a few business days. Although most breast biopsies are not cancer (about 80% are benign), a tissue sample is required to make an accurate diagnosis.

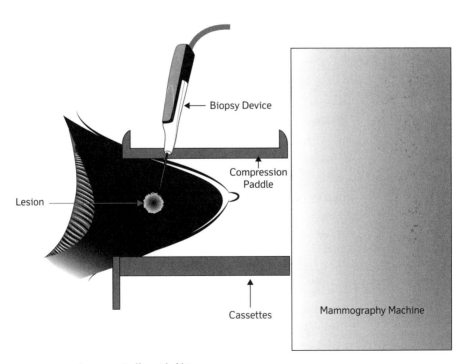

FIGURE 12.2 Stereotactically guided biopsy.

RISKS AND BENEFITS

Stereotactic breast biopsy is reliable and is less invasive, less costly, and less complicated than surgical biopsy according to the American College of Surgeons. It does not require general anesthesia or stitches, and it has a very short recovery period.

Because a small nick is made in the skin, there is a less than 1% risk of bleeding or infection. For women with breast implants, there is a very small risk of implant rupture during the needle biopsy. As with other types of biopsy, there is a remote possibility that the tissue removed will not provide adequate information for diagnosis, in which case a surgical biopsy will be necessary.

WHAT TO EXPECT

This procedure is usually performed in an office setting. The entire process takes about 1.5 hours, but the biopsy itself takes only a small portion of that time. It is advisable to discontinue ibuprofen (Motrin), naproxen (Aleve), aspirin, fish oil, and vitamin E for 5 to 7 days before the biopsy. If you are taking prescription medications that affect blood clotting (e.g., Plavix, Coumadin), contact your physician to obtain permission to stop the medications for 3 to 5 days before the biopsy.

You should wear comfortable clothing; only the top portion needs to be removed. Wearing a sports-type bra for the first 24 hours after the procedure can provide comfort and support. You should eat a light meal before the procedure, and you may drive yourself to the appointment. On arrival, you will be asked to change into a gown and to sign a consent form for the biopsy.

Depending on the facility, the biopsy will be performed while you are sitting or lying down. If sitting, you are seated in a special chair with the stereotactic machine in front of you or at the side of your breast. If lying down, you are asked to lie on your stomach on a specially designed table with your breast placed through an opening in the table. The table is then raised, and the radiologist performs the biopsy from underneath. In either position, the area of concern is compressed with a paddle, as for a mammogram. It is very important that you remain still during the biopsy. Several images are taken, and the computer aids in calculating the exact approach for the biopsy.

The breast skin is cleaned, and the radiologist then numbs the area with a local anesthetic. You will feel a pinch for a few seconds, and then the area will become numb. You should feel only pressure during the biopsy. A small incision is made, and tissue samples are obtained through the biopsy needle. After the samples are taken, a tiny clip is placed to mark the area that was biopsied. Pressure is applied to the biopsy site for a few minutes to prevent bleeding. Steri-Strips and gauze dressing are applied to the incision, but stitches are not necessary. A low-pressure mammogram is done to document placement of the clip.

You will be discharged with an ice pack and written instructions to take home. Acetaminophen (Tylenol) may be used for discomfort. You should avoid lifting or strenuous activity on biopsy day and the next day. Most women resume their normal activities the following day. Tenderness and bruising are common during the first few days after the biopsy.

(Adapted with permission from LuAnn Roberson, RN)

MRI–Guided Needle Biopsy

After reviewing the diagnostic breast images, the radiologist may recommend that you have a breast biopsy to diagnose an area of concern found on the MRI scan. MRI-guided breast biopsy is a minimally invasive, highly accurate procedure that is used to obtain small samples of breast tissue for evaluation (a simplified rendition is seen in Fig. 12.3).

This type of biopsy uses limited MRI images to aid in calculation of the exact location of the tissue to be sampled. As with the diagnostic MRI that found the lesion, it is necessary to inject a small amount of contrast dye into a vein. The lesion accumulates the dye and becomes visible on the images.

The procedure is performed by a radiologist. The tissue samples are sent to the laboratory for evaluation by a pathologist. Results usually are available within a few business days. Although most breast biopsies are not cancer (about to 80% are benign), a tissue sample is required to make an accurate diagnosis.

RISKS AND BENEFITS

MRI breast biopsy is reliable and is less invasive, less costly, and less complicated than surgical biopsy. It does not require general anesthesia or stitches, and it has a very short recovery period.

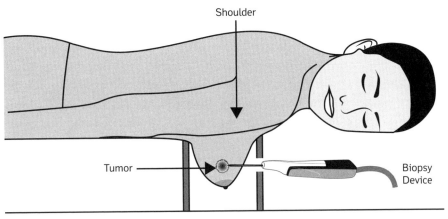

FIGURE 12.3 MRI-guided biopsy.

Because a small nick is being made in the skin, there is a less than 1% risk of bleeding or infection. For women with breast implants, there is a very small risk of implant rupture during the needle biopsy. As with other types of biopsy, there is a remote possibility that the tissue removed will not provide adequate information for diagnosis, in which case a surgical biopsy will be necessary.

WHAT TO EXPECT

This procedure is performed in an office or hospital facility. The entire process takes 1.5 to 2 hours, but the biopsy itself takes only a small portion of that time. It is advisable to discontinue ibuprofen (Motrin), naproxen (Aleve), aspirin, fish oil, and vitamin E for 5 to 7 days before the biopsy. If you are taking prescription medications that affect blood clotting (e.g., Plavix, Coumadin), contact your physician to obtain permission to stop these medications for 3 to 5 days before the biopsy to decrease the potential for bleeding complications.

You should wear comfortable clothing; only the top portion needs to be removed. Wearing a sports-type bra for the first 24 hours after the procedure can provide comfort and support. You should eat a light meal before the procedure, and you may drive yourself to the appointment. On arrival, you will be asked to change into a gown and to sign a consent form for the biopsy.

The biopsy is performed while you are lying on your stomach on the MRI table, which has a breast coil that is specially designed for the purpose of biopsy. Your breast is placed into a space beneath you to hold it in place. A series of pictures are taken with and without contrast to visualize the lesion. This may take 10 to 15 minutes to obtain. The computer localizes the position of the lesion and aids in calculating the exact approach for the biopsy.

The radiologist performs the biopsy from the medial or lateral side of the breast, depending on the location of the lesion. In both cases, the area of concern is only mildly compressed with a paddle, similar to the procedure for a mammogram. It is very important that you remain still during the biopsy.

The breast skin is cleaned, and the radiologist numbs the area with a local anesthetic. You will feel a pinch for a few seconds, and then the area will becomes numb. You should feel only pressure during the biopsy. A small incision is made, and the tissue samples are obtained through the biopsy needle. After the samples are removed, a tiny clip is placed to mark the area that was biopsied. Pressure is then applied to the biopsy site for a few minutes to prevent bleeding. Steri-Strips and gauze dressing are applied to close the incision, but stitches are not necessary. A low-pressure mammogram is obtained to document placement of the clip.

You will be discharged with an ice pack and written instructions to take home. Acetaminophen (Tylenol) may be used for discomfort. You should avoid lifting or strenuous activity on biopsy day and the next day. Most women resume their normal activities the following day. Tenderness and bruising are common for the first few days after the procedure.

(Adapted with Permission from LuAnn Roberson, RN)

Radiologic-Pathologic Correlation

After the radiologist has found a lesion, determined it to be suspicious, proceeded to biopsy, and proved that the targeted lesion has been sampled, is she done? No. The most critical step is the **radiologic-pathologic correlation**. This is a comparison of the pathology findings (i.e., what the pathologist saw under the microscope) with what the radiologist identified on the imaging study (i.e., what the picture showed). Does the pathology finding explain the imaging finding (i.e., **concordant** data), or not (**discordant** data)? Is sampling error possible? Under what circumstances would another biopsy be needed?

Three categories of results can be obtained from the pathology evaluation of a needle biopsy sample. The usual situation is diagnosis of either a clearly benign lesion or a lesion that is clearly cancer. However, there is a third possibility that occurs in a small percentage of cases in which the results show cells that are **atypical** or the particular type of tumor diagnosed has other known implications. In these special cases, the biopsy may lead to a benign result but still require surgical excision.

THE RESULT IS BENIGN

The results are back, and the lesion is reported to be benign (i.e., not cancer). If the lesion was expected to be benign, we are good to go. This is concordant information and explains the imaging lesion. Common pathology diagnoses for benign lesions are fibrocystic changes or sclerosing adenosis (for targeted calcifications), fibroadenoma (for solid tumors), and benign breast tissue or fibrosis (for areas of asymmetry). These examples represent concordant findings. The patient usually gets a 6-month follow-up mammogram to document stability and establish a new baseline after biopsy. However, if the lesion was highly suspicious (i.e., looked like cancer on the image) but the pathology report was benign, the findings is discordant (do not "fit"), and further evaluation with a surgical biopsy is needed.

A few noncancerous conditions, such as granular cell tumor, diabetic mastopathy, and granulomatous mastopathy, can simulate cancer. Surgical consultation is recommended for clinical management to determine whether the patient requires a follow-up evaluation or a surgical excision. These lesions often have clinical presentations that look like cancer (i.e., a firm, hard mass); surgical excision removes the mass and relieves the patient's symptoms.

THE RESULT IS MALIGNANT

If the lesion is malignant, the imaging and pathology results are clearly concordant. At this point, the radiologist must review the case, assess the size and extent of the lesion, and address any other concerns that could affect the patient's care based on the current information. It is helpful to look again at the mammogram and the ultrasound scan to determine whether other lesions have become more suspicious in this new context (i.e., known cancer). Are there other findings that need to be considered? Is the lesion isolated, or is it part of a larger process (e.g., a cluster of calcifications among a larger area of similar calcifications)? Do other areas require biopsy to prove that they are not cancerous before the surgical treatment begins? Has the other breast been evaluated with imaging? Further workup may be needed and may include other studies such as preoperative MRI.

THE RESULT IS BENIGN BUT HIGH RISK

The results from most biopsies are either clearly benign or clearly cancer, but there is a third possibility based on certain diagnoses. These high-risk or atypical findings may be benign but nevertheless may require a surgical biopsy for confirmation. In a small percentage of cases, therefore, it is possible to have a benign needle biopsy result and still need a surgical biopsy to completely exclude malignancy.

Needle biopsy is a sampling procedure, and although it is highly accurate, it takes only pieces of the lesion; therefore, any atypical findings from this type of biopsy should warrant surgical excision (i.e., removal of the entire lesion). *Atypia* means that the cells do not look like garden-variety benign cells under a microscope, but they are not obviously cancer. To ascertain their true nature, they should be looked at in the context of the tissue around them. Taking a contiguous sample (i.e., an intact lump of tissue rather than pieces) allows the pathologist to evaluate the atypical cells, neighboring cells, and surrounding tissue to determine the final diagnosis.

Most of the time, the final diagnosis is that the atypical cells were merely funny-looking normal cells (we all have neighbors like that). However, some atypical findings are upgraded to **malignancy**, usually low-grade **ductal carcinoma in situ (DCIS)**. The distinction is significant. Common diagnoses based on a needle biopsy that warrant surgical consultation for consideration of excisional biopsy are atypical ductal hyperplasia (ADH), atypical lobular hyperplasia (ALH), lobular neoplasia or lobular carcinoma in situ (LCIS), and benign breast tissue with atypia.

Three notable benign lesions may also require surgical excision: papilloma, radial scar, and phyllodes tumor. *Papillomas* are benign tumors that can arise in the breast ducts and are a frequent cause of bloody discharge. They are commonly close to the nipple, and the location of the lesion may give the radiologist a hint that this diagnosis is likely. Although most papillary lesions are benign papillomas, there is such a thing as papillary cancer (Fig. 12.4). Although most cancers are cancers through and through (i.e., cancer is present throughout the sample), papillary cancer cells may be found in only a certain portion of the lesion or scattered throughout the lesion. Because core biopsy is a sampling procedure, the diagnosis of papilloma should warrant surgical excision.

Radial scar is a benign lesion that usually warrants consultation for surgical excision because of its association with intermixed tubular carcinoma. If the lesion is an area of distortion seen on imaging, it will be difficult to follow (observe over time) for changes

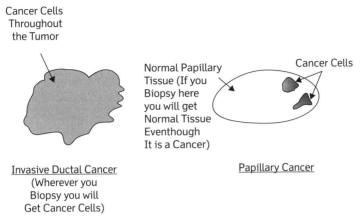

Cancer Cells Throughout the Tumor

Normal Papillary Tissue (If you Biopsy here you will get Normal Tissue Eventhough It is a Cancer)

Cancer Cells

Invasive Ductal Cancer (Wherever you Biopsy you will Get Cancer Cells)

Papillary Cancer

FIGURE 12.4 Papillary cancer compared with other invasive cancers.

because it looks suspicious and is likely to prompt frequent evaluation or workup; therefore, surgical excision may be a less complicated strategy for the clinical management of these lesions and can save the patient a lot of anxiety and grief.

Phyllodes tumors of the breast are benign except for the rare tumor with malignant potential. Even for benign phyllodes, however, the treatment is wide surgical excision (i.e., taking out the lesion plus a thick rind of surrounding normal tissue) to ensure complete removal. Usually, no further treatment is needed.

Cyst Aspiration

Ultrasound-guided cyst aspiration is commonly used to provide symptomatic relief for women with known benign cysts. Women most often request aspiration of cysts because they are palpable or tender. Aspiration deflates the cyst (like a water balloon) and provides relief of symptoms (Fig. 12.5).

Sometimes, it is unclear whether a lesion is a cystic or solid lesion, and diagnostic ultrasound-guided cyst aspiration is needed to determine whether fluid can be retrieved. If fluid is retrieved and the lesion is completely resolved visually on ultrasound, it was clearly a cyst. Because visual confirmation is as accurate as sending the fluid to the cytology laboratory, the fluid can be discarded. If the lesion does not resolve completely, it is likely to be a cyst that has some thick material or debris within it. In this case, the lesion may have almost but not completely resolved after aspiration. The radiologist can decide to use a larger needle and aspirate again, stop and send the material for cytologic analysis, or change the procedure to a core biopsy.

Ultrasound-guided cyst aspiration is a minimally invasive procedure that removes fluid and cellular material from a lump or cyst in the breast. Ultrasound, which does not involve the use of x-rays, guides the radiologist in withdrawing fluid or tissue. Many

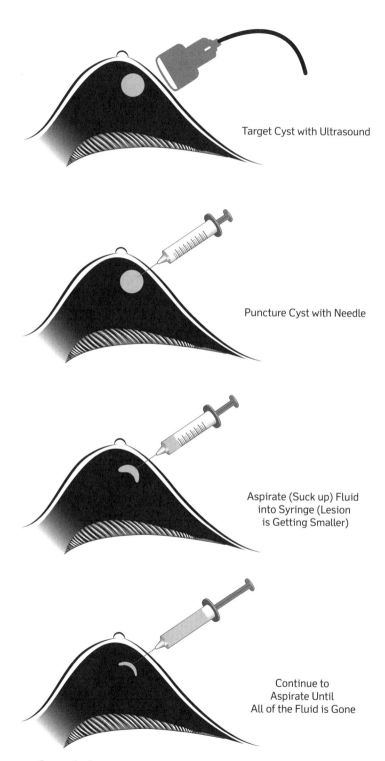

Target Cyst with Ultrasound

Puncture Cyst with Needle

Aspirate (Suck up) Fluid
into Syringe (Lesion
is Getting Smaller)

Continue to
Aspirate Until
All of the Fluid is Gone

FIGURE 12.5 Cyst aspiration.

lumps in the breast are harmless, fluid-filled sacs, but a small percentage of them may contain malignant (cancer) cells. This procedure provides the information needed about the nature of the breast lump.

WHAT TO EXPECT

This simple procedure is usually performed in an office setting. The entire process takes approximately 1 hour, but the cyst aspiration takes only minutes. It is advisable to discontinue ibuprofen (Motrin, Advil), naproxen (Aleve), aspirin, fish oil, and vitamin E for 5 to 7 days before the procedure. If you are taking prescription medications that affect blood clotting (e.g., Coumadin, Plavix), obtain permission from your doctor to stop these medications for 3 to 5 days before the biopsy.

You should eat a light meal before the procedure and should wear comfortable clothing; only the top portion needs to be removed. Wearing a sports-type bra for 24 hours after the procedure provides comfort and support. On arrival, you will be asked to change into a gown and to sign a consent form for the aspiration or biopsy.

During the procedure, you will lie on your back, the area of concern will be scanned by the technologist, and the result will be shown to the radiologist. The radiologist cleans and numbs the appropriate area of your breast with a local anesthetic to prevent discomfort during the procedure. As the area is numbed, you may feel a sting for a few seconds. At this point, one of the following three scenarios will occur:

1. The radiologist inserts a small needle into the cyst and then removes and examines the fluid. If the color of the fluid looks like typical cyst liquid and the cyst collapses when the fluid is withdrawn, the procedure is finished. The liquid is discarded, a Band-Aid is placed over the needle site, and you are discharged. There is no suspicion of malignancy or cancer.

2. The radiologist withdraws fluid from the area and prefers that a pathologist examine it under a microscope. The fluid is sent to the pathology laboratory, and the findings will be reported to you within a few days. A metallic clip may be placed at the time of the procedure to document the location of the aspirated lesion. A Band-Aid is placed over the needle site, and you are discharged.

3. If the radiologist is unable to withdraw fluid because the area appears to be **solid** instead of fluid filled, a small nick is made in the skin, and tissue samples are taken (i.e., biopsy). The tissue is sent to the laboratory for evaluation by a pathologist. A small clip is placed in the breast to mark the area where the tissue was removed. Manual pressure is applied to your breast for a few minutes to prevent bleeding. A low-pressure mammogram is done afterward to document the location of the marker. Steri-Strips and gauze dressing are used to close and cover the site. You are given an ice pack for discomfort along with written

instructions to take home. The biopsy results usually are available within a few business days after the biopsy. Most of the time, no cancer is identified.

Fluid Drainage or Aspiration

If there are suspected pockets of fluid in the breast, radiologists are sometimes asked to drain the fluid for symptomatic relief and sometimes to retrieve the fluid for laboratory analysis to detect cancer cells or assess for infection (i.e., culture to determine the causative organism and determine the sensitivity of the causative organism to various antibiotic therapies). This may be useful for postoperative patients with enlarging or complex seroma cavities, patients with mastitis and an identifiable abscess (i.e., pus pocket), and patients with inflammation and large amounts of fluid surrounding an implant, suggesting infection or rejection.

These procedures are performed in a similar fashion as for cyst aspiration, but a larger-gauge needle typically is used. Rarely are drains needed in these circumstances, although serial drainage procedures may be needed until the inflammation or infection has subsided.

RADIOLOGY CONSULT

Image-guided procedures enable quick, easy, and accurate diagnosis of breast conditions, including confirmation of breast cancer. These procedures have significantly impacted assessment of breast disease and have provided a remarkable advance in women's health.

13

You Do Not Have Breast Cancer

THE VALUE OF A BENIGN EVALUATION

I SEE ON a daily basis the great relief expressed by women when they are told that the outcome of their evaluation is **benign** (i.e., not cancer). Audible sighs and joyful tears are common. When performed within the parameters of legitimate scientific data and the current standard of care, the breast evaluation often is definitive (or as conclusive as possible in the context of current medical knowledge) in making a benign diagnosis and excluding breast cancer.

Many definitive benign diagnoses can explain **abnormalities** found on imaging studies or patient symptoms such as cysts, scar tissue, infection, trauma effects, fibrocystic changes, and hormonal responses. Thus, the benign finding "solves the problem" and answers the clinical question. This is much more reassuring than telling the patient, "We do not see anything." There is something comforting about having the finding or symptom specifically addressed and the reasons for the benign diagnosis explained to the patient and the referring doctor. In many cases, the finding is clearly benign, and the patient and doctor can move on to other things.

It is important to emphasize, however, that no imaging modality is 100% accurate. As knowledge increases and technology improves our ability to diagnose and treat disease, we must not forget that the practice of medicine, although rooted in strong scientific principles, remains an art (as it should be). Outcomes depend on knowledge, technique, equipment, available data, and many other factors.

Outcomes of an evaluation can be **true negatives** (i.e., no disease existed and none was detected), **false negatives** (i.e., disease was present but was not detected), **true positives** (i.e., disease was present and was detected), or **false positives** (i.e., although disease was thought to be present, none was detected). Physical examination, patient history, **mammograms**, and other types of breast imaging studies have different ratios of these four outcomes based on how the examination is performed and its inherent strengths and weaknesses. To optimize detection and minimize error, the radiologist determines the best combination of studies to address the clinical question at hand and reassure the patient that a benign diagnosis based on the evaluation can be trusted. There are many findings of a breast evaluation for which the definitive diagnosis is benign and the radiologist has no concern about the possibility of cancer.

Fibroadenomas (i.e., calcified fibroadenomas) are the most common benign tumors of the breast (Fig. 13.1). When they have chunky, popcorn-like calcifications, they can be diagnosed as benign with no need for a biopsy or follow-up examination. These are sometimes called *degenerating fibroadenomas*.

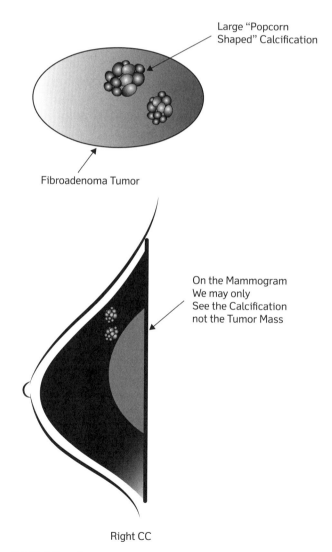

FIGURE 13.1 Calcified fibroadenoma.

Cysts are part of the normal ductal system of the breast. They are outpouchings of a normal duct or ductal unit. They often are single and appear like a water-filled balloon on **ultrasound**. They can be multiple and manifest similar to a cluster of grapes. Ultrasound is the best way to confirm a cyst, and the sonographer uses specific criteria to make this determination (i.e., exclude a solid tumor). Simple cysts look like water on ultrasound and have no internal debris; they appear completely black on the scan. Some cysts contain debris but are still benign. If the sonographer can see swirling debris within the cyst, the finding confirms a fluid medium, and the diagnosis of a benign cyst can be definitively made. If there is any controversy, diagnostic needle aspiration can be performed, or the lesion can be followed with serial ultrasound studies (Fig. 13.2).

Isolated or focally dilated ducts can account for abnormal findings on a mammogram or a **palpable** area of concern for the patient. If the duct is otherwise normal in appearance and there are no tumors within the duct, it can be assessed as a normal, expected finding with no malignant potential.

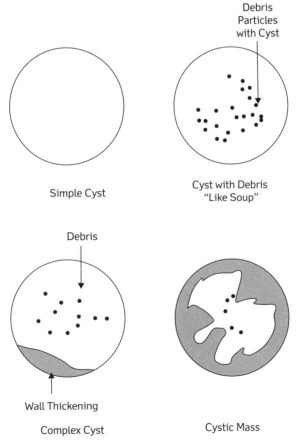

FIGURE 13.2 Types of cystic lesions.

Breast tissue is not a single sheet of tissue; instead, it is separated by ligaments into lobulations that give the breast an undulating feel, like waves in the ocean. Many times, this anatomy explains the feeling of a soft nodularity, even in a **fatty breast**. The patient or her doctor often can feel a fatty lobule as a discrete lump, especially if it lies just beneath the skin (Fig. 13.3). Because I have the advantage of being able to palpate the area of concern while looking with ultrasound to see what accounts for the finding, I often can conclude that the area of the lump is a fatty lobule and not a tumor. A mammogram in this setting also would show fatty tissue in the area, further confirming the diagnosis.

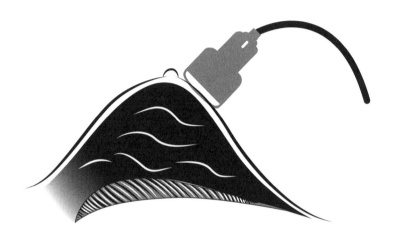

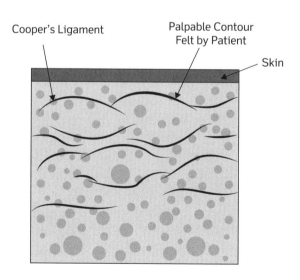

FIGURE 13.3 Fatty lobule manifesting as a palpable lump.

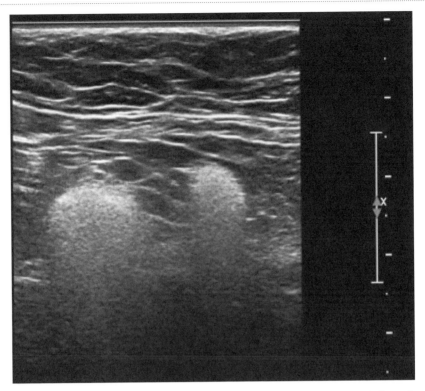

FIGURE 13.4 Appearance of free silicone on ultrasound. (Courtesy of the American College of Radiology)

Free silicone resulting from rupture of a breast **implant** is dense and looks white on mammography. The diagnosis often is evident from the mammographic appearance. However, the ultrasound scan has a classic snowstorm appearance that does not look like anything else and can be used if there is doubt about whether a lesion is a clump of free silicone from an implant rupture or a breast tissue tumor (Fig. 13.4). Ultrasound is usually definitive, but if there is still controversy, **magnetic resonance imaging (MRI)** can be used for confirmation. Although MRI is not usually required, it can be used if additional information about the integrity of the implant is needed.

Hamartomas are segmented pockets of breast tissue that exhibit all of the elements of normal breast tissue. They are sometimes called a "breast within a breast." They have a thin capsule and can have the appearance of a mass, and they are sometimes palpable. If there is fat within the mass, it can be diagnosed as a hamartoma with no follow-up examination or biopsy needed, however there are rare exceptions.

An implant valve is a port through which fluid can be added or removed from a saline breast implant with a needle (Fig. 13.5). It can sometimes be palpated as a lump by the patient or her doctor. It often is located very superficially and can be felt in women who have large implants and thin overlying breast tissue. Real-time ultrasound is the key to

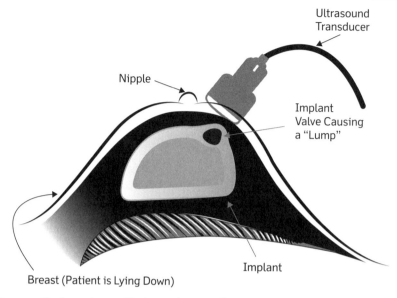

FIGURE 13.5 Implant valve manifesting as a lump on ultrasound.

diagnosis. Because I have the advantage of being able to palpate the area of concern while visualizing the valve on ultrasound, I can often confirm that no breast mass is present that could account for the lump. Making this diagnosis relieves the patient and the doctor from having to follow the lump or get a biopsy. This finding is not an abnormality of the implant and does not need evaluation by a plastic surgeon; it is the normal configuration of the implant that is clinically evident to the patient.

Many implants, especially saline implants, are not filled to capacity so that the breast can look and hang more naturally. The extra room can create implant folds, which can sometimes be felt by the patient (Fig. 13.6). Using real-time ultrasound evaluation, I can often demonstrate that the lump is actually represents the contour of the implant fold.

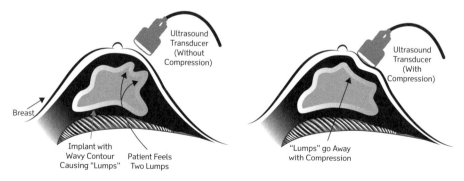

FIGURE 13.6 Implant fold manifesting as a lump on ultrasound.

Compression of the presumed lump with the ultrasound transducer causes the implant to flatten (i.e., reduce), and the artifactual lump disappears on physical examination.

Lipomas, which are fat tumors, have a characteristic appearance on mammography (a gray, fatty density) and on ultrasound (uniformly white or gray density with a thin capsule). When a lipoma can be confirmed as the cause of the palpable lump, the diagnosis is definitive, and no further follow-up or biopsy is needed.

Calcifications are commonly found on mammographic studies. Most calcifications are benign, but cancer also can manifest as calcifications on a mammogram. Sometimes, the calcifications are found within tiny cysts, which can be demonstrated with special mammographic views. This scenario usually occurs when a patient gets a screening mammogram and new or concerning calcifications are seen. She will be asked to return for additional special views (i.e., **recall**), which can include a view from the side. Because calcium is heavier than the fluid within the cyst, it forms a layer on the bottom of the cyst (i.e., milk of calcium), which can be seen as a line on the mammogram. When this occurs, fibrocystic calcifications can be confirmed. This is a benign diagnosis, and no further workup or biopsy is warranted.

Lymph nodes can be located in the breast, most commonly in the upper outer quadrant. Normal lymph nodes can be determined to be benign by their characteristics on the mammogram or on ultrasound (Fig. 13.7). If fat is seen within the center of the lesion and the lesion is well defined, it can be definitively determined to be an intramammary lymph node and diagnosed as benign.

After *trauma* (either accidental or from surgical intervention), the body attempts to heal itself. It can wall off the injured area and form scar around it; this can be seen as an area of fat that has been walled off by a surrounding margin (i.e., an oil cyst) or as thick, chunky calcifications in the area of trauma (i.e., fat necrosis) (Fig. 13.8). In both cases, the appearance is diagnostic of a benign process, and the mass is not cancer.

Sebaceous glands in the outermost layer of skin secrete oily material that lubricates the skin. When the gland's pore is blocked, the thick material cannot exit and accumulates,

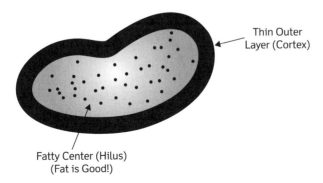

FIGURE 13.7 Normal intramammary lymph node appearance on ultrasound.

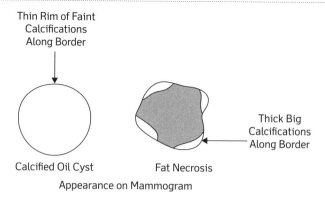

FIGURE 13.8 Mammographic appearance of a post-traumatic oil cyst and fat necrosis.

forming a *sebaceous cyst* that can appear as a superficial breast lump (Fig. 13.9). The small mass beneath the skin is similar to a pimple. On ultrasound, the lesion can be confirmed to be located within the layers of the skin (and not within the breast tissue itself). Often, a track to the skin often can be seen, further confirming the diagnosis. Lesions that are within the skin can be safely determined to be dermatologic in origin and called benign. However, if the patient has a known cancer of any type, the possibility of a subcutaneous **metastasis** (i.e., cancer that has traveled from another site to the area of skin in question) must be considered. If the patient has a known breast cancer and a skin lesion is seen in the lumpectomy site or mastectomy scar, it must be determined whether it represents a local recurrence of the cancer.

Secretory disease is a process of benign inflammation around and within the breast ducts. The result is the appearance of secretory calcifications, which are large, rodlike,

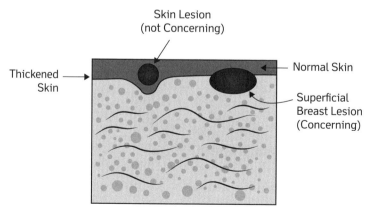

FIGURE 13.9 Sebaceous lesions.

linear calcifications that have a unique and typical appearance. They may be **unilateral**, **bilateral**, or regional in distribution.

Skin calcifications are benign. Additional tangential mammogram views (i.e., views that show the skin on edge) sometimes are needed to confirm the location in the skin. However, they may be readily evident as skin calcificatons on tomographic imaging. and additional recall of the patient is not required.

Skin lesions such as moles, skin tags, keloids, and neurofibromas can project over the breast tissue and appear to be lesions in the breast. For this reason, the technologist marks obvious skin lesions so that the radiologist can correlate the mammographic findings with the physical findings. Tomosynthesis makes this process much easier and the result obvious to the radiologist.

Vascular calcifications that can be confirmed to lie within the walls of blood vessels are benign (Fig. 13.10). They usually are found in arteries but occasionally are seen in veins. If calcifications are seen on a screening mammogram and it is not clear that they are vascular, the patient may be recalled so that additional views can be obtained for further evaluation. The workup includes magnification views that better demonstrate the calcifications, which usually appear as tram-track lines on the mammogram. If they are vascular, they require no further workup or biopsy. Vascular calcifications are a common mammographic finding in older women. Some studies have suggested that arterial calcifications identified in younger women may indicate underlying cardiovascular or renal disease and should be mentioned so that the referring physician can assess the patient for these conditions.

There is another category of findings that can be reliably considered benign based on their appearance and distribution. Radiologists see lots of things on mammograms. If the findings are scattered, multiple, and bilateral and appear similar to one another, they indicate benign systemic processes, not breast cancer, Breast cancer typically does not

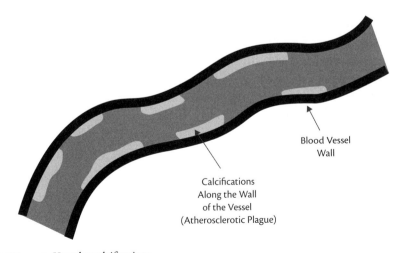

Blood Vessel
Wall

Calcifications
Along the Wall
of the Vessel
(Atherosclerotic Plague)

FIGURE 13.10 Vascular calcifications.

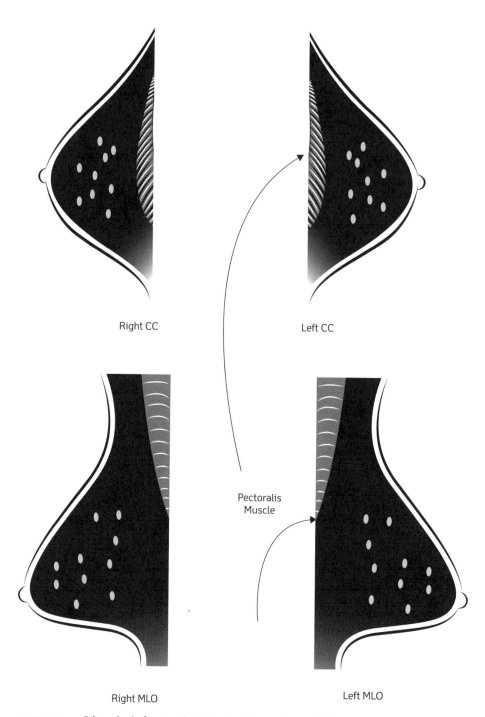

Right CC

Left CC

Pectoralis
Muscle

Right MLO

Left MLO

FIGURE 13.11 Bilateral calcifications (with benign characteristics and distribution).

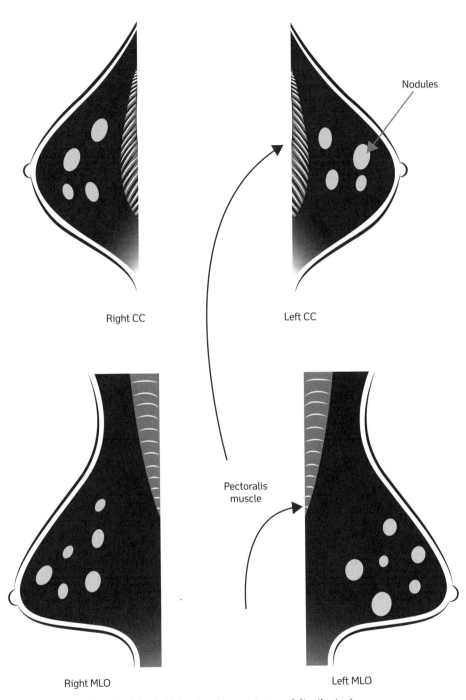

Right CC

Left CC

Nodules

Pectoralis
muscle

Right MLO

Left MLO

FIGURE 13.12 Bilateral nodules (with benign characteristics and distribution).

manifest in such a diffuse manner without other symptoms or findings, and it would be exceeding rare for it to do so bilaterally. Therefore, although there may be many findings, the overall assessment is that the appearance is benign. The fact that the findings are similar to each other is a strong indicator of benign conditions.

Bilateral calcifications that are diffuse, numerous, and usually similar to one another, with no one particular area more concerning than the rest are benign (Fig. 13.11). They are usually relatively symmetric (i.e., similar from one breast to the other). They usually represent diffuse background calcifications in the breast, fibrocystic changes, or sclerosing adenosis.

Bilateral nodularity is another situation in which the diffuse nature of similar findings (i.e., nodules or nodular appearance of the tissue) implies a systemic cause or pattern that is not cancerous (Fig. 13.12). Old films that show stability are particularly useful in this scenario.

Fluctuating fibrocystic changes over time can be demonstrated mammographically. The change usually manifests as multiple masses seen bilaterally. The masses are round or oval and of various sizes. They may come and go (i.e., fluctuate) over time. If the nodules have a favorable appearance and distribution with no overall pattern of worsening, they can be safely called benign, especially if the pattern of changes is decreasing over time or is no more significant than in prior studies.

RADIOLOGY CONSULT

Radiologists have become better at diagnosing a wide range of breast conditions. Knowing what is normal or benign (and having reasons to support that decision) is often as important as knowing what to look for to diagnose cancer.

14

You Have Been Diagnosed With Breast Cancer

THE CRITICAL ROLE OF RADIOLOGY IN TREATMENT

PLANNING AND FOLLOW-UP

A DIAGNOSIS OF breast cancer is immediately life changing for the patient. The best treatment plan with the most favorable outcome is based on knowing as much as possible about the patient's situation to ensure accurate planning. The patient should be involved in every aspect of discussion and decision making. The goal of treatment is to deliver the best outcome possible for the patient and her specific situation. Understandably, the patient has myriad questions: Can I have a **lumpectomy**? Is a **mastectomy** necessary? Will I need radiation therapy? What about chemotherapy? How big is the cancer? Is there cancer in the **contralateral** breast?

The first order of business for the radiologist is to provide imaging data so that the patient's treating physicians can give recommendations based on complete information. The radiologist determines the tumor size and possible spread of disease to the lymph nodes. This may involve re-reviewing the patient's recent **mammograms** or performing additional studies such as **ultrasound** or **magnetic resonance imaging** (**MRI**). Abnormal findings on these studies may require an additional biopsy, which could have important implications for the type of surgery needed. For example, biopsy of **calcifications** in an area of the breast separate from an area with known cancer may prove that the calcifications do not represent cancer and do not need to be considered in the treatment planning, or it may show that they do represent cancer and the surgeon should recommend mastectomy.

Sometimes, this search-and-rescue assessment delays surgery, but the benefit is well worth it because it lessens the chance of unexpected findings at the time of surgery (we do not need surprises here!). Accurately assessing the extent of disease before treatment may decrease the need for additional operations to remove residual (remaining) tumor at a later time and can save the patient and her doctor much grief down the road.

When the Diagnosis Is Made

When I perform a biopsy and the result is positive for cancer, I reevaluate the patient's current imaging (i.e., what has been done to this point) and comment in the biopsy report on the current situation as I understand it. For example, is this a solitary lesion, or are there multiple lesions? What is the size of the lesion? Are the margins well visualized? Is the measured size thought to be an accurate reflection of the tumor size, or is the lesion vague, or with poorly defined margins, or obscured by surrounding tissue? Is the size thought to be underestimated based on the current imaging? Does the lesion have associated benign distortion resulting from surrounding fibrotic changes? Is the actual size overestimated by the current imaging because it represents a small, central finding with surrounding normal tissue being pulled toward it, causing the distortion?

What is the assumed size of the lesion and its distribution (i.e., what area of the breast is involved)? This information helps the surgeon to know how much tissue must be taken out in order to remove all of the cancer plus a rind of normal tissue around it (i.e., negative margins). Does the lesion go toward or involve the nipple, the chest wall, or the skin? These features also aid the breast surgeon in planning and may assist in preplanning for the plastic surgeon, who often is consulted in advance of the operation.

Are the **axillary** lymph nodes abnormal? I routinely assess these regional lymph nodes because they provide valuable clinical information. The treating physicians need to know whether they appear structurally normal or are obviously abnormal and whether there is concern about metastatic disease to this area. The need for biopsy of the axillary lymph nodes before surgery is a matter of debate, but having all of the relevant information before treatment begins seems reasonable. Based on information from a clinical trial, some surgeons recommend not looking at axillary nodes at all. However, radiologists are responsible for evaluating and reporting all information on the films, and it would be suboptimal care and poor protocol not to do so. The surgeon should be made aware of this information, determine its importance for the patient, and make a clinically appropriate decision based on all of the data. Biopsy may be warranted in some situations and not in others, but the decision must be based on knowledge, not avoidance of known data.

Radiologists often recommend performing preoperative breast MRI of both breasts to evaluate the local extent of disease (i.e., the size of a known cancer), multifocal disease (i.e., cancer in tissue adjacent to the area), multicentric disease (i.e., cancer in another part of the same breast), or contralateral disease (i.e., cancer in the other breast). If MRI findings suggest additional disease, a needle biopsy is needed to confirm the tissue diagnosis of cancer.

Some medical authorities are concerned that preoperative MRI increases the likeli-hood that the patient or the surgeon may select a more extensive surgical treatment (i.e., mastectomy instead of lumpectomy) due to **suspicious** results suggesting that the patient has more extensive disease than she really does. Some surgeons do not order MRI for this reason. However, if MRI is used properly and the same parameters are followed as for other imaging modalities (e.g., biopsy is used to confirm the diagnosis), I think it is a very useful tool for many patients. The surgeon and the patient often skip the step of biopsy of additional suspicious areas, then blame the MRI examination for having low **specificity** (i.e., overestimating the extent of disease compared with the final pathologic analysis of surgical samples).

It must be remembered that imaging provides a picture, not a tissue diagnosis. No one goes directly to surgery based solely on a mammographic finding, even if it is highly sus-picious. Needle biopsy is performed preoperatively to confirm the diagnosis. MRI should be treated similarly, and suspicious lesions should be biopsied.

On the Day of Surgery

On the day of surgery, the radiologist often provides needle-guided localization so that the lesion can be accurately removed. The goal is to get all of the known cancer out and be able to prove it. Knowing how radiology fits into the treatment process can make the journey less stressful for the patient.

In most situations, the cancerous tumor has been biopsied preoperatively under imag-ing guidance to confirm that the patient has cancer. It is standard practice in radiology to put a metallic clip in or around the tumor at the time of the needle biopsy. The clip marks the site of cancer and can be seen on mammography (and sometimes on ultrasound scan-ning), even if the lesion is small or not well visualized after biopsy.

Needle localization is done by placing a thin wire through the cancer or by putting more than one wire around the margin of the tumor (i.e., bracketing it) (Fig. 14.1). In the latter situation, the surgeon removes the area between the wires. This method is used if the cancer is located over a larger area and the radiologist wants to ensure that the entire area of concern is removed.

Although the standard method of localizing tumors before surgery is needle locali-zation with a wire, some centers have started using radioactive seed localization of the tumor. This process entails placing a tiny seed containing a very small amount of radio-activity at the site of the cancer. As with wire localization, the seed can be placed in or around the tumor depending on the situation. The benefit of this method is that place-ment can be done before the day of the surgery (i.e., 1 to 5 days in advance), making the day of surgery is less hectic because the patient does not need to visit the radiology department on that day. In the operating room, a Geiger counter is used to detect the radioactivity of the seed, and this guides the surgeon to the area of the tumor that needs

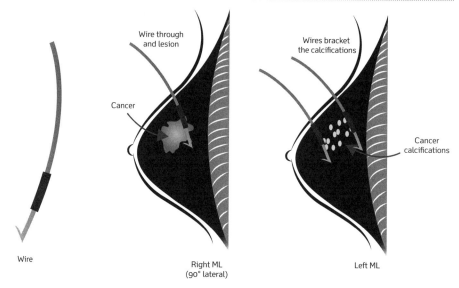

FIGURE 14.1 Needle localization and bracketing.

to be removed. Additionally, newer methods of seed locatizations are being used with seeds that require infrared or magnetic detection devices. The advantage of these newer methods is that the seed is not radioactive and the seed can be placed up to 30 days before the surgery.

Assessing the status of the axillary lymph nodes is standard in breast cancer surgery because cancers that spread outside of the breast usually go first to the underarm lymph nodes and does so in a reliable sequence. The sentinel node is the first lymph node (or the first few nodes) to which the breast vessels drain. Drainage then predictably proceeds toward the deeper-level lymph nodes. It does not skip to the second-level lymph nodes without first going through the sentinel node or nodes.

Having information about the sentinel node is essential. If the result is negative (i.e., no cancer in it), the rest of the axillary lymph nodes can be assumed to be cancer free, and the patient may require no additional surgery in the underarm area. This means that the patient can avoid the full operation (i.e., axillary dissection) that would be needed in some instances to remove the diseased nodes but can lead to long-term debilitating complications i.e., a painful, swollen arm.

Identification of the sentinel node can be accomplished by two techniques. The preoperative injection method is performed by a radiologist or a surgeon. A low dose of radioactive material is injected around the nipple of the affected breast or around the cancer. The radioactive material travels to the underarm and sticks to the sentinel lymph nodes, which allows the surgeon to localize them with a Geiger counter and remove them. In the second method, the surgeon injects blue dye under the nipple or around the cancer at the time of surgery and visually tracks the dye as it moves toward the underarm (intraoperative method). The surgeon then resects (i.e., cuts out) the lymph nodes that have intense blue dye accumulation. Both methods may be used. Both have good success rates, and the method chosen depends on the preference and experience of the surgeon.

As surgery day continues, the time comes for the surgeon to remove the cancer. The cancer has been localized in some manner by the radiologist, and the surgeon uses this guidance to cut out the cancer along with a rind of normal tissue around its entirety to achieve negative margins. This approach ensures that all of the cancer that was visible on the imaging films is removed. It is preferable for the specimen to be removed as one contiguous piece of tissue (i.e., not cut into small pieces) so that the tumor can be seen and assessed relative to the edges of the specimen.

An x-ray film of the tissue is frequently taken at the time of the surgery (Fig. 14.2). The radiologist reviews the film immediately to confirm that the tumor has been removed. The needle biopsy clip is an indicator that the area that was biopsied (and proved to be cancer) has been included in the specimen and is now out of the patient's breast. If the clip is not in the specimen, the radiologist notifies the surgeon. They then come up with a plan to localize the lesion based on knowledge of the case and what has been done so far.

Assuming that the tumor is seen on the specimen film, the tissue surrounding the known cancer is also investigated. Is the whole tumor included in the specimen, based on size and appearance? Do I see the whole lesion that was targeted? Is there concern that some tumor is still left in the breast? How close to the margin of normal tissue is the tumor? Is there adequate normal tissue around the edge (e.g., no tumor cells within 1 cm of the cut), or has the tumor been cut close to the margin or even transected (sliced through)? The need to answer these questions is the reason the specimen radiograph should be assessed at the time of surgery, while the patient is still in the operating room. If additional tissue needs to be taken out, it can be done during the same surgery. Having a system in place and timely communication of these findings by the radiologist to the surgeon can facilitate proper treatment and save the patient a second operation to achieve adequate margins. A little bit of extra time up front can save a lot of headaches later.

First Imaging After Surgery

The first imaging examination after treatment provides as a new baseline appearance against which the radiologist can compare all subsequent films for change or stability. It establishes what the tissue looks like after the treatment.

Most initial imaging is performed 6 months after surgery to give the breast time to heal so that the compression needed for the mammogram can be used and so that adverse postoperative or postradiation changes (e.g., inflammation) are not so acute (Fig. 14.3). This produces a better image for the radiolotist to review. If a lumpectomy was done for calcifications and the patient is scheduled to have radiation therapy, I recommend performing a mammogram as soon as the patient is able to comply (1 month is usually

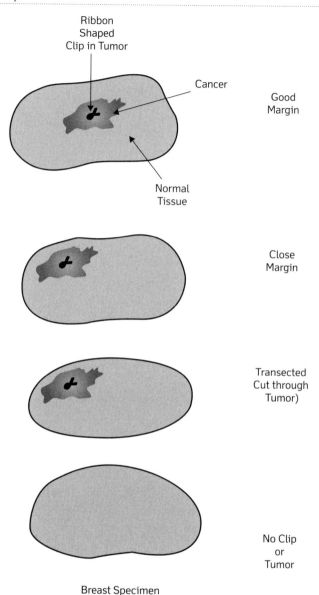

Ribbon
Shaped
Clip in Tumor

Cancer

Good
Margin

Normal
Tissue

Close
Margin

Transected
Cut through
Tumor)

No Clip
or
Tumor

Breast Specimen

FIGURE 14.2 X-ray image of a surgical specimen.

adequate) to confirm that all of the cancerous calcifications were removed. If calcifications are present, indicating that there may be remaining cancer in the breast, the patient may be taken back to surgery to remove the known cancer before radiation therapy is started.

In the typical case, the patient returns 6 months after surgery for a diagnostic evaluation of the breast on the side of the lumpectomy. Her treatment history is important

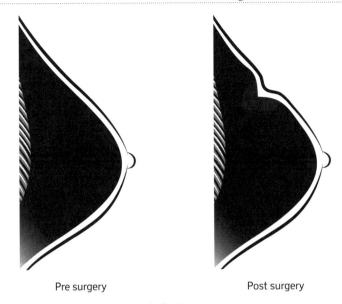

Pre surgery   Post surgery

FIGURE 14.3 Initial mammogram obtained after lumpectomy.

because it affects the radiologist's interpretation of the images. The surgery site should be identified and marked on the skin for the mammogram so that the distortion or cavity on the film clearly correlates with the surgery and is not interpreted as a new suspicious finding. The radiologist needs to know whether the treatment involved brachytherapy (i.e., internal radiation therapy using a balloon or rods placed in the breast at the site of the lumpectomy cavity) or whole-breast irradiation (i.e., external beam irradiation of a large portion of the breast, not just the lumpectomy site) because these procedures result in different imaging appearances.

The usual postoperative changes include distortion at the site of the lumpectomy, distortion at the site of the axillary surgery, inflammatory changes or swelling in the tissues surrounding the surgery site, and postradiation changes. If the patient had brachytherapy, the lumpectomy site may have a large oval mass mimicking the shape of the balloon device. If the patient had whole-breast irradiation, there is usually diffuse puffiness of the tissue evidenced by a strandy, fluffy appearance of the lines of breast tissue. This is described in the radiologist's report as trabecular thickening. Both types of radiation therapy typically result in skin thickening, which may be localized or may involve the whole breast, depending on the length of treatment and what portion of the breast was treated.

The diagnostic workup at this time usually involves a mammogram and ultrasound evaluation (Fig. 14.4). Because I usually do my own ultrasound scanning, I can clearly identify the surgical site, correlate the treatment history with the imaging findings, address any concerns the patient may have, and relay my findings to the patient at the time of the evaluation. She can leave the facility knowing what I know about her case.

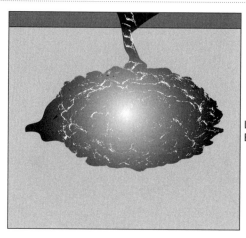

Lumpectomy Cavity
Extends to Skin

FIGURE 14.4 Ultrasound study after lumpectomy.

Knowing the history is essential to accurately interpret the images. First, the radiologist must confirm that the cancer has been removed (i.e., the previously seen tumor is no longer seen and the clip that was placed during the needle biopsy has been removed). During the operation, the surgeon places a new clip (or clips) in the lumpectomy site to clearly mark the area where the surgery was performed. Because this is the area of the previous cancer, it will be monitored closely.; The surgical clip can be seen on subsequent mammograms, and the radiologist should not mistake it for a needle biopsy clip indicating residual tumor.

Next, the imaging findings are correlated with the known history (i.e., in relation to expected posttreatment changes). The radiologist assesses for any new and concerning findings that may indicate interval development of cancer at the original site or elsewhere in the breast.

Subsequent Imaging After Treatment

After the first postoperative evaluation, the patient returns in 6 months for another diagnostic examination. This evaluation is performed bilaterally because it is time to look at the other breast (i.e., we do not want to miss the annual assessment for that breast). Mammography and ultrasound examinations are usually performed, and the images are compared with the first posttreatment films that were obtained 6 months earlier.

I assess the images for stability or improvement of findings. The lumpectomy site may look smaller and have less tissue strandiness around it, indicating healing. Trabecular thickening of the tissues may be reduced, and there may be less skin thickening as the acute inflammation from the radiation therapy improves. What I do not want to see is progression of these findings, which can indicate recurrent disease or complications of treatment. An example is increasing density (seen as whiteness on images) or increasing size of the lumpectomy cavity.

Depending on the imaging findings, drainage or a biopsy may be indicated to determine whether there is recurrence of disease. There may be new calcifications at the site that look worrisome, and if it cannot be determined whether they represent a new cancer or early fat necrosis (i.e., healing calcifications), a **stereotactic** biopsy may be indicated.

The Special Case of Preoperative Chemotherapy

If the patient begins chemotherapy before surgery, multiple follow-up tests may be needed to determine how she is responding to it. This is called *neoadjuvant chemotherapy* (as opposed to adjuvant chemotherapy, which is given after surgery). Chemotherapy, which is prescribed and administered by a medical oncologist, is given intravenously (i.e., in the veins) through a catheter to deliver the medicine throughout the body and destroy the cancer cells in the breast and elsewhere (e.g., liver, brain, bones, bloodstream). An example is the drug Herceptin, which is an antibody engineered to preferentially attack tumors that have HER2-type receptors on the surface of cancer cells. The drug decreases the size of the targeted tumor and does not affect other cells in the body. The response can be swift, with a significant decrease in tumor size or tumor eradication as seen on imaging.

The test used to follow the progress of these patients depends on the best way to see the tumor. Sometimes it is mammography, and sometimes it is ultrasound or MRI. The radiologist's role is to evaluate whether the known cancer is getting bigger, getting smaller, or staying the same during the preoperative chemotherapy. This tells the medical oncologist whether the treatment is working. If it is working and is significantly shrinking the tumor's size, the patient may not need a mastectomy as initially thought and could have a lumpectomy instead. Tumor progression indicates that the chemotherapy is not effective. The time intervals chosen for follow-up and management decisions in such cases are determined by the medical oncologist. The radiologist's role is to assist with the available imaging methods needed to help the oncologist treat the patient.

RADIOLOGY CONSULT

Radiology plays an important role after a cancer diagnosis is made. Useful information from imaging is provided at many steps along the treatment path. Management is greatly improved by close collaboration between the radiologist and the treating physicians (e.g., surgeon, radiation oncologist, medical oncologist). I am a great fan of the multidisciplinary conference, in which the entire team gets together to discuss cases and give advice and recommendations regarding our particular specialties, although getting on the phone and talking to the referring doctor sometimes is just as efficacious. There should be easy access and liberal communication between the breast radiologist and the treating physicians at all points during the patient's treatment.

V

Other Considerations

If anything is sacred, the human body is sacred.

WALT WHITMAN

15

Special Cases

PREGNANCY, LACTATION, BREAST IMPLANTS,

LYMPHOPROLIFERATIVE DISORDERS

AND MALE BREAST CANCER

A FEW SUBSETS of patients require special mention. They are pregnant patients, lactating patients, patients with implants, patients with abnormal lymph nodes and male patients.

Pregnancy

Imaging for pregnant women always elicits questions and hesitation because of concern about the damaging (teratogenic) effects of radiation on the fetus. Because the amount of radiation to breast tissue from a **mammogram** is extremely low and the dose to the fetus is negligible, it is safe for a pregnant woman to have a mammogram. That being said, this remains a source of confusion for many patients.

The American College of Radiology (ACR) provides guidelines for imaging evaluations of women who are pregnant or potentially pregnant. The ACR states, "Mammography can be performed at any time during pregnancy. Radiation exposure to a conceptus from a properly performed screening mammogram is inconsequential."

In the setting of pregnancy, the patient's concerns are taken very seriously. Although the radiologist may feel comfortable proceeding with a mammogram, the patient may not. For example, she may believe that she would be exposing her baby to harmful radiation if she has a mammogram. I review the risks and benefits of mammography with the patient and make an assessment based on her individual situation. Can I make an accurate diagnosis using other imaging modalities such as ultrasound? How strongly does mammography affect my evaluation? Would I be harming my patient by not doing a mammogram and possibly delaying a diagnosis of breast cancer?

Ultrasound is the first line of assessment for pregnant patients. If the findings are unremarkable or show an obviously benign lesion, I am comfortable with deferring the mammogram, especially if the physical findings are not suspicious. In this setting, I request that the patient return after delivery to complete the evaluation with mammography. Chapter 19 provides a thorough discussion of safety issues in breast imaging.

Lactation and Breastfeeding

Lactating women also are frequently given conflicting information about their eligibility for breast imaging studies. They have no additional risk from mammograms compared with their nonlactating, age-matched counterparts. Breast milk is not affected, and no cessation in breastfeeding is required. The limitations usually are based on the patient's comfort level concerning the breast compression that is necessary for a technically adequate image. I recommend that women who are lactating should breastfeed or pump their breast immediately before the evaluation to decrease the amount of engorgement, thereby allowing for optimal compression and improved visualization of the tissue.

Breast Implants

Another controversial imaging situation involves women with breast **implants**. Implants might have been placed to achieve **reconstruction** after mastectomy or **augmentation** for cosmetic reasons. Each of these situations has imaging limitations and other considerations. Knowledge about the type of implant and the relevant history (e.g., replacements, rupture) impacts care and the accuracy of image interpretation.

For patients who have had a mastectomy and reconstruction with implants, routine mammographic screening of the reconstructed breast has not proved cost-effective or clinically useful. Physical examination is an adequate replacement.

For a woman who has undergone augmentation with implants, several factors may alter the workup compared with that for someone who does not have implants. First, a routine screening mammogram for an augmented breast requires at least eight (not just four) images. The additional views are in the same projection as the standard views, but the implant is displaced so that the native breast tissue can be adequately compressed and evaluated.

The position of the implant in front of the chest wall muscles (i.e., **pre-pectoral**) or behind them (i.e., **retropectoral**) may determine the amount of native breast tissue that can be visualized. Implants are seen as big white masses on a mammogram, and they can obscure a significant amount of breast tissue. Breast tissue that is not seen cannot be evaluated, and abnormalities (sometimes cancers) may exist in these obscured regions but without being detectable even with technically optimal images. Although implant displacement views can be quite good and the techniques for positioning are improving all the time, it is rare to have no limitations in imaging in the presence of implants.

Lymphoproliferative Disorders

Occasionally, radiologists are able to diagnose lymphoproliferative disorders by evaluation of the mammogram. These systemic primary lymph node conditions usually present as bilateral enlarged dense lymph nodes in the axillary regions (Figure 15.1). The intramammary lymph nodes may be enlarged as well. These disorders may be non cancerous such as the result of an inflammatory arthritis or malignant such as chronic lymphocytic leukemia (CLL) or lymphoma. I have diagnosed several cases of lymphoma that were not previously known to the patient or her physician (clinically occult) by the mammographic appearance. Of course, biopsy of the abnormal lymph node is required to confirm the diagnosis.

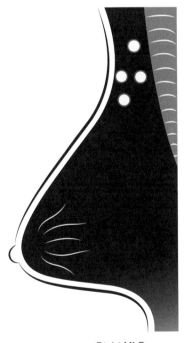
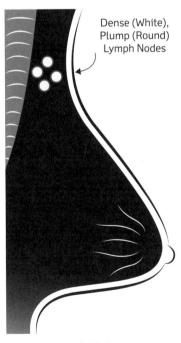

Dense (White), Plump (Round) Lymph Nodes

Right MLO   Left MLO

FIGURE 15.1 Bilateral abnormal axillary lymph nodes.

Male Patients

Male breast cancer, although rare (1% of cases), is a true entity and usually manifests as a **unilateral** lump. The workup is identical to that for a woman. Fortunately, we are seeing more men (with the support of their primary care physicians) who are comfortable being evaluated for breast-related symptoms at a breast center. Men can get a perfectly acceptable mammogram.

The most common breast abnormality in a male patient is gynecomastia, which is enlargement of the glandular tissue of the breast (Fig. 15.2). It is most frequently

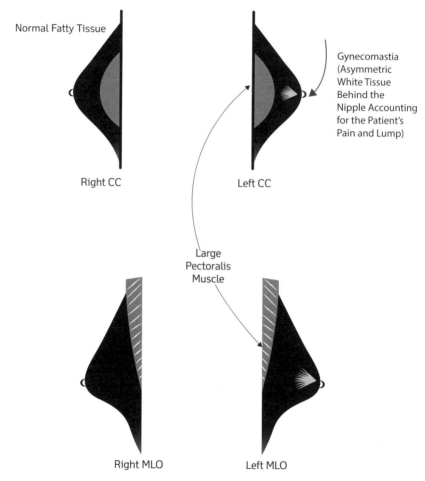

FIGURE 15.2 Male gynecomastia.

encountered in teenage boys and elderly men, and it often is attributed to shifts in the relative amounts of testosterone and estrogen. The patient usually has pain and a lump behind the nipple of one breast (i.e., unilateral gynecomastia).

Gynecomastia is a benign condition and requires no treatment. Causes include medications (e.g., steroids, heart medications, antidepressants), street drugs (e.g., marijuana) and alcohol, and certain diseases (e.g., overactive thyroid, kidney failure, liver cirrhosis). The referring physician should review the patient's health history to determine whether any of these factors are causative. If gynecomastia is the result of medication use, the patient and his doctor can determine whether changing to another medication is worthwhile. Although the reason for gynecomastia often is not evident (i.e., idiopathic cases), the condition is benign and is not associated with an increased risk of breast cancer. No imaging follow-up is needed.

RADIOLOGY CONSULT

I challenge women to do their due diligence before getting augmentation implants, at least to the degree that they would for getting a new hair stylist. They should ask a lot of questions. Informed women can make a logical, appropriate decision to get breast augmentation, but many times the decision is not based on a comprehensive investigation by the patient. This level of inquiry would be prudent for any woman considering breast augmentation, but it is especially consequential for women with high-risk profiles (e.g., strong family history of breast or ovarian cancer). There is no need to make the process of finding a cancer any more challenging than it already is.

16

How Does Your Report Get to You and Your Doctor?

NO NEWS IS NOT NECESSARILY GOOD NEWS

THE ADAGE THAT "no news is good news" is wrong in the context of medical testing, especially for breast imaging. Although most results are **negative** (i.e., **benign** diagnosis), lack of communication or lack of documentation to prove communication of the findings has served as the central theme in malpractice lawsuits claiming that a delayed diagnosis resulted in loss of the best chance for treatment outcome.

The responsibilities of the **radiologist**, the ordering physician, and the patient are reviewed in this chapter (highlighted terms are defined in the Glossary). Tips are offered about how to optimize the communication process and ensure the proper exchange of information so that delays are minimized.

The communication process can be short-circuited in several ways. The radiologist may have found a lesion and dictated a report but without any documentation that the report was received by the patient or communicated to the referring doctor. The referring doctor may have ordered the examination without following up to get the results or without reviewing the radiologists report, which was filed and never acted on. The patient may have had the examination without following up to get the official results from the ordering physician, assuming that if the findings were suspicious, someone would contact her; or, she may have been told of the results but was too afraid to return for another appointment. Each of these scenarios has been the focus of lawsuits, resulting in real harm to patients and real damage to physicians.

The Radiologist and Radiology Facility

The process of reporting is mandated for radiology institutions performing mammograms to minimize miscommunication or noncommunication of all results, whether good or bad. The **Mammography Quality Standards Act (MQSA)** mandates direct communication of results by the radiologist or radiology facility to the patient in the form of a lay letter, which explains the results in understandable language.

For a **mammography** facility to be in compliance, there must be in place a notification system or process of communication regarding significant findings, such as for screening patients who need to return for additional evaluation or those for whom a biopsy was recommended who have not returned for the procedure. Although protocols can be specific to the particular facility, most involve sending the patient the lay letter and having a breast center staff member call the patient to schedule the appointment or procedure. If a patient does not respond to attempts at communication, there must be a system in place to document attempts to contact her, including possibly sending certified letters and communicating the noncompliance to the referring physician.

The Referring Physician

Once a test is ordered. it is the responsibility of the ordering physician to have a system in place to document that the procedure was actually performed and the results of the test were made available, reviewed, and, if appropriate, acted on. Simply reviewing those reports that happen to come across the desk is not enough. There must be a system to track what has been ordered and what the results are. This is the referring physician's obligation as the legally responsible medical provider.

The Patient

Although the radiologist and the referring physician have legal and ethical responsibilities to a patient, the ultimate responsibility, from a practical standpoint, must be shouldered by the patient because it is she who bears the consequences of any delay in diagnosis or treatment of a serious disease. A patient knows that she had a test and should be interested enough in her own care to follow-up on the results. Patients should not assume that someone else will take responsibility for their care.

It is not unreasonable to ask a patient to follow-up on her test results with the facility or with her doctor. After consulting a radiologist for an assessment and recommendation, the patient should make the decision to comply and follow through or to decline further care. An informed refusal is an appropriate response and can resolve the issue.

RADIOLOGY CONSULT

The end game for communication of results is to ensure that significant results are acted on and that the patient gets the care and treatment she needs. If we all take our roles seriously, there will be fewer instances in which noncommunication or miscommunication leads to harmful or potentially harmful outcomes for patients. Communication errors by the radiologist or the referring physician are certainly unintentional, which why it is important for any practice to have backup protocols in order to minimize these types of communication mishaps.

17

Patients' Questions About the Imaging Evaluation

LEARNING MORE CAN SAVE YOUR LIFE

"MY DOCTOR SAYS that my breasts feel normal, but I think that I feel a lump—what should I do?" "My doctors have always told me that I have fibrocystic breasts—what does that mean?" "How often can I have a screening mammogram?" "Will the mammogram rupture my implants?" "Will my insurance pay for an additional diagnostic mammogram even though I just had my screening mammogram last week?" These and other questions about breast imaging are answered in this chapter.

Ten Common Questions

Ten frequently encountered questions from patients about the imaging evaluation in my practice are the following (provided courtesy of nurse navigator LuAnn Roberson, RN, BSN, CN-BN):

1. Can I have ultrasound every year and not have to undergo the pain and radiation exposure associated with a mammogram?
   Answer: **Mammography** is the best screening tool for detection of breast cancer (highlighted terms are defined in the Glossary). It is the only test that has been proven to decrease death rates from breast cancer as a result of early detection. A mammogram is almost always the first step. **Ultrasound** is a good helper test, but it is not by itself a good stand alone screening tool.

2. My doctor says that my breasts feel normal, but I think that I feel a lump—
   what should I do?

   Answer: Your concerns about your **self breast examination (SBE)** are just
   as valid as your doctor's reliance on a **clinical breast examination (CBE)**.
   If you think you feel a lump that is concerning, address the issue with your
   doctor, who can order a diagnostic breast evaluation (i.e., mammogram and
   ultrasound).

3. My doctors have always told me that I have fibrocystic breasts—what does
   this mean?

   Answer: Many referring providers describe the diffuse nodular feel of the
   breast tissue as *fibrocystic*. I have seen this term for a lumpy pattern used for
   patients with completely fatty breasts as well as for women with dense breasts
   and all patterns in between. For **fatty** and **average**-density breast tissue,
   palpation of the breast lobules (which are segmented by ligaments) reveals a
   lumpy pattern. In dense and very dense breasts, it is the firmness of the tissue,
   more than the lobulations, that typically accounts for the findings on the
   CBE. However, most women do not have true fibrocystic changes which are
   demonstrated on imaging by, multiple **cysts**, clusters of cysts, and dilated ducts
   throughout the breast tissue and are evident on mammography, ultrasound, or
   magnetic resonance imaging (MRI).

4. If I have mammograms year after year, will the radiation do damage to my
   breast over time and cause cancer?

   Answer: No. The amount of radiation that you receive from a mammogram is
   miniscule compared with almost all levels used in medical imaging and even
   with background environmental sources. Mammography is very safe and has
   the great benefit of detecting early breast cancers. Starting at 40 years of age
   and having yearly mammograms over a lifetime results in a very low cumulative
   dose exposure. It is well below what I as a radiation worker am allowed in 1
   year. No studies have demonstrated the develpment of breast cancer from the
   low doses of radiation used in medical imaging.

5. Because I do not have cancer in my family, can I reduce my mammograms to
   every few years?

   Answer: No. Only 25% of women diagnosed with breast cancer have a known
   family history or other risk factors; 75% of breast cancers are diagnosed in
   women without known family history or other risk factors. The two biggest
   risk factors for getting breast cancer are gender (being a woman) and age
   (getting older). For average women, the most lives are saved by having annual
   screening mammograms starting at age 40 years.

6. I do not have cancer, and I am thinking about getting **implants**. Can the **radiologist** still get good pictures afterward, and will the mammogram rupture my implants?

   Answer: Special "implant-displaced" mammographic views are performed for women with implants to provide good visualization of the breast tissue. Although the implants do cover up some areas of the breast tissue, good mammographic pictures can still be obtained, depending on how mobile and pliable the implants are. Results can be limited if the implants are hard and encapsulated and therefore difficult to move out of the way. The amount of breast compression needed for a mammogram is not enough to rupture an intact implant.

7. I have always had cysts, and I think I have a new one. Should I wait until my yearly mammogram time to check it out?

   Answer: No. If you have a new lump, you should address the issue with your doctor as a new finding. Your doctor should refer you for a diagnostic evaluation and not wait for the routine screening examination. Having had cysts in the past does not mean that a new lump will also be a cyst. The new lump should be assessed based on its own merits.

8. If my lump is cancer, will poking it with a needle for a biopsy cause it to spread?

   Answer: No. Image-guided **needle biopsy** is a safe and effective method of diagnosing breast diseases, including breast cancer. Biopsy using this method does not result in spread of the tumor to other parts of the body or change in the stage of the cancer.

9. Will my fibroadenoma turn into cancer over time if it is not removed?

   Answer: No. Fibroadenomas, the most common benign tumors of the breast, do not turn into cancer. They can be stable, increase or decrease in size, or rarely resolve completely. After being confirmed as fibroadenomas, they do not require removal unless they are rapidly growing or are producing symptoms (e.g., palpable lesion, tenderness).

10. I am told that I need an additional diagnostic mammogram even though I just had my screening mammogram last week. Why do I need another mammogram, and why should I have to pay for it when the tech obviously did not do it right the first time?

    Answer: A properly performed screening mammogram study is composed of standard views with good positioning (to see as much of the breast tissue as possible on the film) and good technique (to ensure that elements of the breast tissue are well demonstrated). The role of the technologist is to give the radiologist a good picture of the breast. The radiologist interprets the film by looking at it for abnormalities. If an **abnormality** is found on your screening mammogram, you will be recalled for additional investigation of that finding. The diagnostic mammogram is a problem-solving tool that includes special views. It may include magnified images or images from a different angle to determine whether the area is concerning. (Similarly, if you have an abnormal finding on a standard electrocardiogram, the cardiologist may order a Holter assessment that monitors your heart for 24 hours). The initial test looks for abnormalities in general; the additional diagnostic test seeks to identify the specific problem.

Other Interesting Questions

1. I have a lump but did not tell the technologist at the time of my screening mammogram, and the report I got says that everything is fine. If there were a problem, it would have shown up, right?

   Answer: Not necessarily. A screening mammogram is based on the assumption that the patient has no known problems or no significant new problems. You need a diagnostic (problem-solving) mammogram and ultrasound scan to look specifically at the area of the lump. What you have had so far is not adequate. Keeping information from the staff and not providing an accurate history can delay detection of a cancer or confirmation of a benign finding.

2. I received a letter stating that I need to come back for a technical **recall**. What does that mean?

   Answer: Although the **radiologic technologists** strive to perform the best examinations they can and review the films before sending the patient home from the facility, patients occasionally must be called back to get better films to complete the test. A technical recall means that the radiologist has reviewed the technical and positional aspects of the films and believes that they are not optimal or need improvement. In these instances, interpretation may be limited, and the radiologist wants the best films possible to read. We do not want to miss an important finding because the film is substandard. Reasons for a technical recall include not having enough posterior tissue on the picture (which could cause a lesion in this area to be missed because it is not on the film), skin folds overlapping a portion of the breast tissue (the lesion may not be identified because the skin covers it up), motion artifact (because the image looks fuzzy, calcifications may not be visible), or an artifact on the cassette (which could appear as an abnormality within the breast even though it is not real). Because these flaws may cover up or exclude a potentially important finding, the radiologist requests that the films be repeated. There is no additional charge for repeat imaging due to technical recall because it is only a completion of the initial screening study. This is different from a recall for diagnostic imaging, in which there is no technical issue with the images but, instead, a finding on the screening mammogram that needs to be looked at more closely.

3. How long will I be radioactive after my mammogram?
   Answer: You are not radioactive. X-rays used for mammograms travel *through* the breast to produce the image that is captured on a film cassette or digital system. They do not accumulate in the body. There is no radioactivity in the breast as the result of a mammogram.

4. Should I stay away from young children after a mammogram because I have had radiation?
   Answer: Because there is no accumulation of radiation in the breast from a mammogram, no precautions are needed around young children or any other persons.

5. Do mammograms pop the cancer and make it spread?
   Answer: No. The amount of compression from a mammogram does not "pop" or break open a cancer. Even the intervention of biopsying the lesion with a needle does not make the cancer spread within the breast or to other parts of the body. Mammograms and other breast tests are used to diagnose cancers so that they can be treated. They do not cause the disease or spread the disease.

RADIOLOGY CONSULT

It is my hope that the information in this book can clarify many of the questions women have about the process and implications of the breast imaging workup. Being better informed can increase confidence in the process, decrease anxiety, and ensure better care for patients.

Breast Imaging Meets the Outside World

18

Medicolegal Issues and Liability

CAN BREAST IMAGING SURVIVE THE LIABILITY CRISIS?

THE BREAST CANCER Awareness Campaign has without question increased interest in breast health and advanced the associated sciences. However, it has also inadvertently harmed breast imaging as a practical matter because of the common misperception that all breast cancers can be cured if discovered early and that any other outcome must be the result of malpractice and not the natural history (i.e., progression) of the disease. The medical profession, in its zeal to entice women to participate in screening, has promoted the benefits of imaging without a similar public education about the complexities in diagnosis and the inevitable outcomes of this sometimes devastating disease. At times, this has produced substantial detrimental effects for those practicing in the field. A realistic portrait has been slow in coming to the public forum.

From a layperson's perspective, all bad outcomes must be someone's fault or the result of a medical error along the way. In the litigious setting of the today's American culture, this misperception has seriously confounded the problem. Many doctors perform significantly more risky procedures than breast imaging (e.g., neurosurgery, cardiac surgery), with far more potentially serious bad outcomes (e.g., immediate death), but malpractice lawsuits for breast cancer and breast-related issues is near the top of the list in terms of the number of claims and in the size of monetary awards. This is a direct result of the emotionally charged nature of the topic.

Radiologists have become the most commonly sued physicians in breast cancer cases because of "loss of best chance" claims. The perceived and real liability is a psychological deterrent to many radiologists' willingness to read mammographic films. The high risk of malpractice suits makes fewer radiologists willing to interpret the imaging examinations and fewer residents (i.e., radiologists in training) interested in pursuing fellowships or specialized training. The result is a decreased pool of highly trained radiologists experienced in breast imaging. Moreover, **mammography** services often are a money-losing venture, or at best a break-even aspect of a practice, creating another obstacle to providing accessible and affordable breast health care (highlighted terms are defined in the Glossary). Some practices cannot afford to provide the service. The result is fewer locations for women to receive services, longer wait times to get an appointment, greater distances to travel, and fewer facilities performing the high-tech procedures that are sometimes required, such as 3D mammography (Tomosynthesis) or **magnetic resonance imaging (MRI)**.

What is even more damaging is that jurors (i.e., those making the decision of culpability) have no basic understanding of how radiologists find 240,000 breast cancers among the 44 million mammograms they interpret every year in the United States. This makes a sympathetic jury more likely to deliver a verdict in favor of a patient whose cancer was not identified by the radiologist, regardless of the evidence. As in any field, there are bad doctors in radiology, but most radiologists who perform breast imaging are extremely committed and conscientious about patient care. I do not know of any radiologist who has intentionally decided to do substandard work. Many malpractice decisions are not based on understanding of the actual circumstances but instead on understandable empathy for the patient and poor comprehension of the science and professional practice of breast imaging. Only perfection is permissible, and it is an unattainable standard.

RADIOLOGY CONSULT

The current litigious environment for radiologists involved in breast imaging is growing increasingly harsh. Tort reform has been slow and controversial. Some (mainly attorneys) say that liability is the price of doing business, but for many doctors, the emotional and financial costs are too high. Radiologists have become intimidated by this fractured medicolegal environment. Eventually, although the capacity to find curable cancers is greater than ever before, we may find that many fewer radiologists are willing to run the risk of interpreting the studies. This would be a tragic state of affairs.

Take calculated risks. That is quite
different from being rash.

GEORGE S. PATTON

19

Safety Issues in Mammography and Breast Imaging

ASSESSING THE RISK-BENEFIT RATIO

Mammography

Patients and referring physicians are concerned about radiation safety in mammography, mostly regarding pregnancy (i.e., potential harm to the fetus) and the possibility of radiation-induced cancers. Use of the term *safe* in any clinical setting must be understood in the context of the benefit compared with the risk. Safety is a matter of taking appropriate actions to limit the risk to a level that is well justified by the benefit. Mammography has well-established, substantial benefits that must be considered when discussing its risks.

All ionizing radiation is potentially harmful. There is no safe level of radiation exposure per se. However, all levels of risk must be compared with the benefits derived from the activity associated with the exposure. For example, the miniscule risk of radiation exposure during mammography is far outweighed by its benefits.

The American College of Radiology (ACR) has issued guidelines for women who are pregnant or may become pregnant in regard to imaging services. The ACR states, "Mammography can be performed at any time during pregnancy. Radiation exposure to a conceptus from a properly performed screening mammogram is inconsequential."

Most data on radiation-induced malignancies are extrapolated from populations such as survivors of the Chernobyl nuclear accident in 1986 or the atomic bombing of Japan in World War II. These groups received a one-time, high-dose exposure (>500 mSv). They are very different from today's patients who may receive repeated, low-dose exposures (0 to 100 mSv) from medical imaging procedures. No studies have shown a direct cancer risk for the low doses used in medical imaging.

There are valid concerns about radiation exposure in medical imaging, of course. The most significant dose concern involves **computed tomography (CT)**, because there has been an exponential rise in the use of CT in the past 20 years (highlighted terms are defined in the Glossary). Use of CT has produced tremendous advancements in medical care leading to substantial benefits for patients, but concerns about the cumulative dose received from multiple examinations are legitimate. These concerns are aggressively and responsibly addressed by the ACR and the Radiological Society of North America (RSNA) in their Image Wisely Campaign. Ultimately the risk of a miniscule radiation dose from mammography is inconsequential compared with the benefit of possible detection of early breast cancer and consequent decreased **mortality** in the population.

Each view obtained during a **digital** mammogram is associated with a dose of about 0.1 to 0.3 mSv; most complete examinations involve less than 1.2 mSv. If a woman were to receive an annual screening mammogram from age 40 to 80 years, her lifetime cumulative dose would still be significantly less than what I as a radiation employee can safely receive in 1 year (50 mSv). When **tomosynthesis** (i.e., three-dimensional mammography) is added to the two-dimensional (2-D) examination, the total dose per examination is still less than 2.5 mSv. If a C-view examination (i.e., synthetic reconstruction of 2-D images replacing the standard digital 2-D images) is performed, the dose for the overall study is reduced by almost one half.

The goal of all medical imaging is to provide a way to confirm or exclude disease while making the patient's radiation exposure "as low as reasonably achievable" (ALARA). Technologic advances and dedicated specialists in the field of radiology continue to look for improved ways to provide high-quality images with even lower radiation exposures for patients.

The potential received dose or exposure from imaging needs to be evaluated in the context of the annual exposure we all receive from background radiation in the natural environment, which is about 3 mSv according to Edward Hendrick. In the same article another medical physicist, Michael O'Connor, has stated, "The cumulative effect of background radiation over your life is far, far greater than any of these medical procedures."

As with all medical imaging that involves radiation exposure, common sense and clinical usefulness of the study should be considered. Any decision about whether to proceed with an examination should be based on the clinical circumstances of the patient, but mammography remains one of the safest examinations in radiology.

Sonography

After mammography, breast **ultrasound** is the most commonly used test in breast evaluations. The images are produced by sound waves. Ultrasound uses no radiation, is safe to use in pregnancy, and is the test of choice for patients younger than 30 years of age.

Magnetic Resonance Imaging

Breast **magnetic resonance imaging (MRI)** does not use ionizing radiation (such as x-rays or gamma rays). Instead, it uses strong magnets that cause temporary changes in the cells that can be detected and transformed into images of breast tissue. The magnetic environment of the MRI room is not harmful to a fetus. However, the intravenous contrast dye that is used for all breast MRI examinations (except those done to evaluate **implants**) should not be used during pregnancy because it passes through the blood-brain barrier and is detrimental to the fetus (absolute contraindication). In a pregnant patient with breast cancer, other approaches for evaluating the extent of disease must be used. This may include a decision to proceed with treatment based on the available information and perform an MRI after the baby has been delivered.

Molecular Imaging

Nuclear medicine studies are another method of looking for tumors of the breast. The two most common techniques are **breast-specific gamma imaging (BSGI)**, also known as molecular breast imaging (MBI), and **positron emission mammography (PEM).** Like mammography, these studies use ionizing radiation. Unlike mammography, in which x-rays are sent *through* the patient to produce the image, nuclear imaging involves administration of the radioactive material to the patient through injection or other means; the material collects in areas of activity (e.g., cancer), and radiation is emitted from the patient. A special gamma camera is used to detect the radiation activity coming from the patient, and a picture is produced from the resulting data.

The dose of radiation in molecular imaging studies is considerably higher than in digital mammography (e.g., 5.9 to 9.4 mSv for BSGI, 6.2 to 7.1 mSv for PEM). For this reason, these tests are not typically used for screening purposes. They are primarily used in diagnostic situations, such as when cancer has already been diagnosed and use of molecular imaging to search for other cancers in the breast can provide a more accurate assessment and better treatment options for the patient. These studies can be performed in patients with pacemakers and in those who cannot have preoperative MRI. In these situations, the doses are acceptable because the real benefit far outweighs the potential risk.

Other Considerations

Although it is not specifically a breast imaging issue, it is important for CT imaging to be used judiciously in young women because of the radiation dose to the breast tissue. Use of a breast shield during the CT examination can reduce the effective dose by 25% to 50%.

RADIOLOGY CONSULT

Mammography involves an extremely low, almost inconsequential radiation exposure. As with any test, common sense should prevail, and the clinical usefulness of the study should be considered. Any meaningful assessment requires that the risk be assessed in the context of the benefit. There is substantial benefit for mammography, which decreases deaths from breast cancer, and the risk is minimal with the doses currently used. Because mammography is one of the safest tests in medical imaging, women should not "throw out the baby with the bathwater"!

20

The Breast Density Discussion

INFORMATION VERSUS NOTIFICATION

TWENTY-FOUR STATES HAVE enacted legislation mandating that patients be notified if their breast consistency is dense based on the **mammographic** appearance. This information is provided to the patient as an additional comment in the postexamination lay letter that she receives as mandated by the Mammography Quality Standards Act of 1992 (MQSA). This chapter discusses the origins of the breast density controversy along with its merits, limitations, and potential harms as it relates to the clinical care of patients and as a legislative mandate by state governments.

The **density** of a woman's breast depends on the relative amounts of fatty tissue and dense tissue that make up the composition of her breasts. Fatty tissue appears gray or transparent on mammographic films, whereas dense tissue has an opaque, white appearance (Fig. 20.1). Some women have breast tissue that is almost entirely fatty, some women have tissue that is almost entirely dense, and there are many variations in between. The composition (i.e., relative amounts of fatty and dense tissue) and pattern (i.e., distribution of tissue types) of each woman's breast is unique. (See Topics in Breast Imaging: Terms About Breast Tissue Composition.)

If the amount of dense tissue on a mammogram is between 50% and 74%, the breast is described as being **heterogeneously dense** (highlighted terms are defined in the Glossary). If the amount of dense tissue is greater than 75%, the breast is described as having **extremely dense** tissue. Both of these categories are considered dense for the purposes of this discussion and for notification purposes (Box 20.1). Approximately 40% of women have mammograms that indicate heterogeneously dense breasts. Approximately 10% of women have mammograms indicating extremely dense breasts. This means that about one half of the women receiving mammograms have dense breasts.

Radiologists classify breast density using a 4-level density scale:

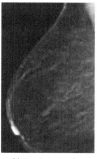 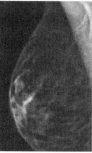 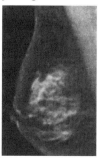 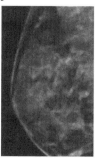

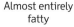

| Almost entirely fatty | Scattered areas of fibroglandular density | Heterogeneously dense | Extremely dense |

FIGURE 20.1 Mammograms showing four density types. (Courtesy of the American College of Radiology.)

Currently, 24 states have laws mandating direct written patient notification of mammographic breast density in the form of a lay letter. Connecticut was the first state to implement mandatory notification (in 2009) as a result of the advocacy of Nancy M. Capello, PhD (see her website at areyoudense.org). The state of Arizona requires that patient lay letters for women with dense breast tissue contain the following statement:

> Your mammogram indicates that you have dense breast tissue. Dense tissue is common and is found in 50% of women. However, dense breast tissue can make it more difficult to detect cancer in the breast by mammography and may also be associated with an increased risk of breast cancer. This information is being provided to raise your awareness and to encourage you to discuss with your health care providers your dense tissue and other breast cancer risk factors. Together, you and your physician can decide whether additional screening options are right for you. A report of your results was sent to your physician.

BOX 20.1

IMPLICATIONS OF TWO TYPES OF BREAST DENSITY

1. Heterogeneously dense tissue may obscure small masses (affects 40% of women).
2. Extremely dense tissue reduces the sensitivity of mammography (affects 10% of women).

Society of Breast Imaging Policy and Position Statements on dense breast and whole breast ultrasound

Two other states, Maine and Utah, have made recommendations suggesting but not requiring mandatory written notification. Ten states have pending legislation regarding the issue of breast density notification to patients. However, only four states currently mandate insurance coverage for annual screening breast **ultrasound** examinations (i.e., complete survey of the breasts in an asymptomatic patient). This is significant because ultrasound is the most commonly suggested supplemental test (in addition to their screening mammogram) for these women to detect cancers not evident on mammography.

The density notification campaign has been accomplished through public advocacy and not from the radiology community. This is primarily because there has been no long-term research experience or data to establish a standard recommendation for which supplemental examinations should be performed, how often, and under what protocols. Although the density discussion is important as an impetus to spur greater awareness, mandatory notification has made the topic more confusing for all involved, including the patient.

As a woman, I would assume that if a state legislative body mandates notification of some information, the information is significant and proceeding through life without it could be dangerous. I would also assume that some type of action needs to be taken— otherwise, why would the notification have been mandated? However, there are at present *no established recommendations* within the field to give women. Although advocacy has increased awareness, the mandatory notifications have confused the entire screening issue and left many patients, referring physicians, and radiologists to make decisions about a patient's care based on less than optimal data.

As a practical matter, radiologists are tasking a patient who has very little information about the implications of mammographic density and a referring physician with no expertise in imaging with determining whether supplemental studies are required in addition to the mammogram. Further, we are assuming that they can chose the appropriate supplemental test (e.g., tomosynthesis, ultrasound, **magnetic resonance imaging [MRI]**, **breast-specific gamma imaging**) and the appropriate testing intervals. The local radiologist may be consulted and may have personal or practice preferences, but no standardized protocols have been established in the field of radiology as a whole. For this reason, recommendations vary from facility to facility and from region to region.

Unlike the extensive scientific data showing a clear survival benefit for annual screening mammograms starting at 40 years of age, there are as yet no data to support a survival benefit for the use of additional tests in women with dense breasts and an average population risk. Women with identical histories and risk profiles may receive different recommendations and different types of imaging. Some variations in management choices are likely to result from insurance coverage, or lack of coverage, of additional imaging studies.

All that having been said, what does the density of breast tissue actually mean, and why is it relevant to the patient, the referring physician, the radiologist interpreting the films, or anyone in the state legislature? What are the implications for breast health screening and breast cancer detection? It is well established in breast imaging that increased density of the breast tissue can reduce the **sensitivity** of mammography, especially for extremely dense breasts. This makes sense because many of the abnormalities (including cancers) that radiologists look for appear white on a mammogram, and dense tissue likewise appears opaque white. In these cases, radiologists have the difficult task of looking for white lesions on a white background.

The presence of dense tissue is also an independent risk factor for breast cancer. A woman with dense breasts has a greater chance of getting breast cancer than a woman who has fatty breast tissue, even if their histories are otherwise identical. Dense tissue is metabolically active tissue and confers two to four times the relative risk of developing a breast cancer compared with fatty breast tissue.

All women have at least a 1 in 8 (12%) lifetime risk of developing breast cancer by 95 years of age. Dense breast tissue increases that risk by a factor of 1.2, effectively resulting in a 1 in 7 lifetime risk, or 15%. These figures should be compared with those for someone with a very strong family history of breast cancer, who may have a lifetime risk of 20% to 25%, and for someone with a *BRCA* gene mutation, which may increase her lifetime risk to between 40% and 80%.

Does the increased lifetime risk in women with dense breast tissue (i.e., from 1 in 8 to 1 in 7) change what doctors do from a practical standpoint? Is a relative risk significantly above the average risk enough to routinely add supplemental imaging for one half of the women in this country undergoing annual testing? If so, what additional test should be done? How often should it be performed? Should it be performed by the radiologist, the **ultrasound technologist**, or an automated system? Are there enough resources and manpower to provide the service if all of the women who are eligible seek to have the test done?

We know what to do for women who have dense breasts and *gene mutations*. They get genetic counseling and screening with ultrasound and MRI in addition to mammography, usually alternating mammography with ultrasound and MRI every 6 months. Some of these women elect to have prophylactic mastectomies. According to the American Cancer Society recommendations of 2007, women with an increased risk above 20% meet the criteria for adding annual MRI to their annual mammogram screenings.

What should be done for with women with dense breasts who have *additional risk factors* but a lifetime risk below 20%? It is reasonable to add a survey ultrasound examination in this instance. The radiology literature suggests that screening whole-breast ultrasound is capable of detecting cancers that cannot be found by mammography (some studies demonstrate detection rates for additional cancers similar to those of screening mammography). These studies were performed in academic institutions with protocols for examinations performed by experienced radiologists (although in most imaging centers across the country, studies are performed by technologists). However, ultrasound is readily accessible in most imaging centers and is relatively inexpensive. Questions remain about how the ultrasound evaluations are performed and whether insurance allows for ultrasound to be performed as a screening test.

For women with dense breast tissue and *no additional risk factors*, I do not think that routine ultrasound is currently indicated as a standard annual examination. Unlike screening mammography, screening breast ultrasound has not been shown to decrease death rates from breast cancer. The American College of Obstetrics and Gynecology (ACOG) does not recommend screening ultrasound for density alone if there are no additional risk factors. Further studies have shown that more early cancers can be found with screening ultrasound but a much larger number of **false-positive** findings also are generated, resulting in a large and unacceptable number of unnecessary breast biopsies according to the American College of Radiology Imaging Network (ACRIN) 6666 Trial. If screening ultrasound is used in this population, I think it should be reserved for those 10% of patients with very dense breasts.

Women with dense breast tissue and *average risk levels* should comply with the recommendation of annual screening mammography commencing at age 40 because data from all organizations demonstrate that this protocol saves the most lives by detecting cancers earlier than they otherwise would have been. I emphasize getting a mammogram every year. Mammography is most beneficial when it is done annually because radiologists can recognize subtle changes when imaging films are compared with prior studies, and this provides the best chance of finding the cancer at the earliest possible time. Both recommendations vastly improve a woman's chance of surviving cancer.

It is also reasonable to suggest that women with dense breast tissue should optimize their mammographic experience by selecting the "optimal" mammogram, **tomosynthesis**. Tomosynthesis adds considerable information for the radiologist and has been shown, along with the experience and training of the radiologist, to detect more invasive cancers than traditional two-dimensional mammography alone and to reduce the number of unnecessary breast biopsies generated by screening ultrasound studies.

The original question remains: What more, if anything, should be done for women with dense breast tissue? Mammography is by far the best screening test for the detection of breast cancer in women with all breast densities. It makes sense to optimize the benefits of mammography by having annual mammograms and by choosing three-dimensional mammography (i.e., tomosynthesis) if it is available. If the patient has additional risk factors, a survey ultrasound study may find additional cancers not detected by mammography. The studies with the best accuracy for screening ultrasound have been those performed by radiologists. However, in most community settings, the technologist, rather than the radiologist, performs screening ultrasound scans. Automated systems that require neither a radiologist nor a technologist to physically perform the study are being developed and are used in some settings, but they have high rates of **false-positive** results and still require some oversight by the technologist and a directed evaluation by the radiologist.

More information on this topic can be found at http://densebreast-info.org/, which is an educational website that addresses questions about breast density. It is particularly useful because its contributors and reviewers are medical experts, ensuring that the information is medically accurate and clinically useful. Recommendations in this chapter were drawn from several sources that also can provide information for patients, such as the Society of Breast Imaging policy and position statements on dense breast and whole breast ultrasound (http://www.sbi-online.org/RESOURCES/PolicyPositionStatements. aspx), the American College of Radiology's *ACR BI-RADS Atlas* (see Bibliography) and statement on breast tomosynthesis (https://www.acr.org/About-Us/Media-Center/Position-Statements/Position-Statements-Folder/20141124-ACR-Statement-on-Breast-Tomosynthesis), and websites addressing the topic of dense breasts such as breast-density.com and areyoudense.org.

> RADIOLOGY CONSULT
>
> Although women are now empowered with knowledge of their breast density, radiologists have no consistent plan for managing the care of women based solely on breast density. Medical research has not produced clear recommendations for radiologists to follow in this instance. Research is ongoing, but until more data are forthcoming, I think we are putting the cart before the horse.

Topics in Breast Imaging

TERMINOLOGY 101

HAVE YOU EVER read a Radiology report and still had no idea of what it said? This outline of Topics in Breast Imaging will clarify the most common and confusing terminology in breast health. Unfamiliar terminology hinders your ability to understand what is being explained or recommended. It is one of the reasons that your perception of what was said does not always correlate with what the doctor thought was conveyed. Obviously, any dialogue that conveys information that you must first understand and then apply to your health care decision making is critical. Simply understanding that a *negative* examination is "good" and that a *positive* finding is "bad" is a huge step in the communication process. Full understanding of the context and implications of information and findings is required if you are to be truly an informed patient.

The terms used by those within a field help them to succinctly and effectively communicate information. Based on agreed conventions, certain words and phrases have a specific meaning within the context of a particular field of study. There is no need for exhaustive explanation because everyone knows what that term means and what it implies when used by practitioners. For instance, according to *Dorland's Illustrated Medical Dictionary*, an <u>adenoma</u> is defined as a "benign epithelial tumor in which the cells form recognizable glandular structures or in which the cells are clearly derived from glandular epithelium." Yet, 86 different types of adenomas are listed, each with a different meaning and implication depending on variables such as where the lesion is located, what it produces, its activity level, or the type of study being performed. There are nuances within the field that express specific or implied meaning depending on who reports the term and the context in which it is reported.

This section has been included to clarify the fundamental breast health terminology so that the discussions within the book will be understandable and make sense. The common nomenclature in *The Breast Test Book* is broken down into easy-to-understand, commonsense terms so that you and your doctor are speaking the same language. Please be aware that these terms are defined according to how they are used in the field of breast imaging; they may have a different meaning if used in a different context.

There are two basic ways to use this section: (1) find the topic of interest to your situation and use the information as a general overview, or (2) refer back to this section and use it for clarification while reading other chapters in the book. The following categories of topics in breast imaging are covered in this section:

A. Terms about **Imaging Results**
B. Terms about **Cancer**
C. Terms about **Breast Imaging Studies and Equipment**
D. Terms about **Procedures and Biopsies**
E. Terms about **Biopsy Results**
F. Terms about **Reporting Your Past Surgical History**
G. Terms about the **Frequency of Imaging**
H. General terms about **Imaging Findings**
I. Terms **Useful for Understanding Mammography**
J. Terms **Useful for Understanding Breast Ultrasound**
K. Terms **Useful for Understanding Breast MRI**
L. Terms about **Lesion Location**
M. Terms about the **Distribution of Findings**
N. Terms about **Conclusions and Recommendations**
O. Terms about **Breast Tissue Composition**
P. Terms about **Physical Examination of the Breast**
Q. Terms about **Breast Surgeries for Benign Conditions**
R. Terms about **Cancer-Related Breast Surgeries**
S. Terms about **Statistics**
T. Terms about **Personnel**

A. Terms About Imaging Results

Negative—No abnormalities were identified; there is no evidence of cancer, based on certain imaging criteria and the ability of that particular examination to detect the finding. The degree of accuracy for detecting breast cancer is different depending on the examination; for example, a negative screening mammogram has a much higher degree of certainty than a negative screening breast ultrasound study when assessing for breast cancer.

Benign—Not malignant; showing no evidence of cancer. There are notable findings, but they have imaging characteristics that are favorable and are not believed to be cancer.

Probably benign—Very likely to be benign; there is an extremely low likelihood of malignancy. In the assessment of a mammographic finding, it implies a greater than 98% probability that the finding is benign and that biopsy can be safely deferred with appropriate follow-up (surveillance).

Suspicious—The finding is concerning for malignancy; the degree of the concern can vary. Biopsy is recommended for suspicious findings so that tissue can be obtained and sent to the laboratory for confirmation. The concern for cancer may be termed mildly, moderately, or very suspicious.

  Mildly suspicious—The possibility of cancer is low, but the finding is concerning enough to warrant biopsy. The benefit of finding a small cancer (one that is likely to be in an early stage and may be curable) is greater than the risk of the procedure. The outcome is statistically more likely to be benign than cancer.

  Moderately suspicious—The likelihood that the lesion is cancer is approximately as great as the likelihood that it is benign. The finding has features of both benign and malignant conditions; biopsy is warranted for further evaluation.

  Highly or very suspicious—There is a high probability that the finding is cancer. The finding has the features of cancer, and biopsy is recommended to confirm. There are a few benign conditions (e.g., granular cell tumor) that can also have malignant features and simulate cancer on imaging.

B. Terms About Cancer

Malignant—Refers to a broad category of disease that includes carcinomas and other processes; a cancer, especially one with the potential to cause death. In breast imaging, the term is generally used interchangeably with Carcinoma (the most frequently encountered type of malignancy). A breast cancer can start from breast tissue cells (i.e., primary breast cancer), or it can represent a metastasis to the breast from another source such as lymph nodes (lymphoma), lung, stomach, or ovary.

Carcinoma—A malignant new growth made up of breast cells tending to infiltrate the surrounding tissues and give rise to metastases.

DCIS (Ductal carcinoma in situ)—Earliest form of breast cancer; the cancer is fully contained within the straw-shaped breast duct and theoretically has had no chance to spread elsewhere in the body. Likely curable if treated appropriately.

Invasive—Refers to any breast cancer that has broken through the straw-shaped breast duct or is infiltrating (invading) into the surrounding tissues. These cancers theoretically may have invaded adjacent blood vessels or lymphatic vessels, so metastatic disease is a possibility; the statistical likelihood of metastatic disease can be estimated based on factors including tumor size and grade.

Ductal—Invasive ductal carcinoma (IDC), the most common type of breast cancer. It arises from the ductal elements in the breast tissue. The pathologist can determine the type by review of the tissue under the microscope and by performing special tests and stains in the laboratory.

Lobular—Invasive lobular carcinoma (ILC), the second broad group of invasive cancer encountered; less common than IDC. This type of cancer is difficult to diagnose clinically and also notoriously hard to detect on mammography because its growth pattern is vague and it may not form a mass; it may manifest as subtle changes in density (whiteness) on a mammogram or merely as decreasing size of the breast.

Multifocal—More than one cancer (from the same process) is present, yet they are either adjacent to one another or near one another and are still contained within a 25% wedge (quadrant) of the breast. Lumpectomy is possible based on imaging; other clinical factors need to be considered as well.

Multicentric—More than one cancer is present, but they are separated from one another by some distance and are in different portions of the breast (i.e., not in the same quadrant of the breast). Lumpectomy may not be possible, and mastectomy may be required.

Unilateral—On one side only; cancer is present in one breast (either left or right), but not in both.

Bilateral—On both sides. The presence of cancer in both breasts may represent two different types of breast cancer.

Ipsilateral—Refers to the "same" side of the body relative to a known lesion; opposite of contralateral. For example, if a patient has a known right breast cancer, a new finding in the right breast would be described as occurring in the ipsilateral breast.

Contralateral—Refers to the "other" side of the body relative to a known lesion; opposite of ipsilateral. For example, if a patient has a known right breast cancer, a new finding in the left breast would be described as occurring in the contralateral breast.

Synchronous—The simultaneous occurrence of two events; in regard to breast cancer, two or more cancers are diagnosed in one or both breasts at or about the same time. They may represent two different types of cancer (e.g., one may be an IDC, and the other may be an ILC).

Metastatic—Cancer in the breast has spread outside the confines of the breast, to lymph nodes or other organs or to the opposite breast via blood vessels or lymphatics. This is what accounts for mortality associated with the disease.

Mortality—Death directly related to a particular disease. In the case of breast cancer, the mortality rate varies based on tumor size, tumor grade, distant metastasis, and type of treatment (i.e., surgery, chemotherapy, radiation therapy).

C. Terms About Breast Imaging Studies and Equipment

Mammography—Imaging modality in which x-rays are sent through the breast tissue to produce a flat (two-dimensional) representation of the breast. In this image, fatty areas appear gray, and dense areas appear white. Compression of the breast is necessary for adequate interpretation. The associated dose of radiation is very low.

> **Film-screen**—Traditional method of acquiring mammogram films. A cassette containing a piece of film captures the image; the film is then run through a processor and developed (as in darkroom photography). The resulting image is evaluated by the radiologist.

> **Digital**—Images are acquired and displayed using computer-based technology; this allows for manipulation of the images by the radiologist, which may result in better interpretations and fewer recalls. Found by a large, multisite study to have an advantage over film-screen images in younger women and in women with dense breasts. Currently the standard of care in most facilities.

> **Tomosynthesis (3-D mammography)**—Multiple, thin-slice mammographic images are acquired, allowing the radiologist to see inside the depths of the breast, similar to a CT examination. Instead of two images per breast, there may be 150 to 200 images, providing a considerable amount of additional information and a higher confidence level for reporting a study as benign. As the "optimal" mammogram, this modality is useful for all breast densities, but especially in women with dense breasts. In the screening population, 3-D mammography offers at least a 30% decrease in recalls. Lesions that are real are seen better, and some are seen only on the tomographic images, leading to increased detection of small invasive cancers, which is the goal. As the person who interprets the examination, I can say that if I were queen, everyone would have a 3-D screening mammogram!

Ultrasound—Also called Sonography. Sound waves are used to generate an image. An ultrasound technologist (or the radiologist) puts a probe on the skin and can see inside to the tissue. It is primarily used to determine whether a lesion is a cyst (fluid) or solid (tumor). Commonly used as an adjunct ("helper") technique to better characterize a mammographic finding or to assess for palpable lesions. Ultrasound increasingly plays a role as an supplemental screening examination (in addition to screening mammography), especially in women with extremely dense breast tissue.

MRI (Magnetic resonance imaging)—Uses extremely strong magnets to cause changes in the tissue (not harmful) so that images can be produced; for breast tissue evaluation, contrast dye containing gadolinium is injected. The way in which the tissue responds to the magnets, the timing of the images, and the amount of dye enhancement provide information about the makeup of the tissue that can be useful in detecting cancers. MRI can be used as an adjunct ("helper") modality along with the standard imaging (mammography and ultrasound) or as a screening tool in high-risk patients.

PEM (Positron emission mammography)—A molecular imaging examination in which uptake of a glucose (sugar)-based tracer chemical is used to detect activity in cancer cells. Cancer activity can be identified before it is visually detectable as a structure or mass.

BSGI (Breast-specific gamma imaging)—A molecular imaging test in which a radioactive tracer is injected into the patient; the radioactive material preferentially accumulates in tumors (both cancers and some noncancer tumors), and a special gamma camera is used to detect the "activity" in the tumor cells and produce an image.

CAD (Computer-aided detection)—A type of computer software program that can be applied to either film-screen or digital mammogram images. The program scans the film to detect and mark any of the findings that it has been programmed to find. This alerts the radiologist to examine the area closely. The Radiologist is then responsible for noting the finding and determining its significance. Because CAD does not have the ability to compare old films or incorporate the patient's known surgical and biopsy history, approximately 90% of the marks are appropriately ignored. CAD is most useful for detecting small clusters of calcifications that may be missed at first glance.

D. Terms About Procedures and Biopsies

Percutaneous—Means "through the skin"; refers to biopsies performed with a needle, which requires a puncture through the skin into the breast.

Cyst aspiration— A procedure in which very thin needle is inserted into a cyst (or focal fluid pocket), similar to puncturing a water balloon, and the fluid is pulled back into a syringe. In breast imaging, this is done under ultrasound guidance to direct the needle into the cyst and to confirm that all of the fluid has been removed. The risk is similar to that of a blood draw.

FNA (Fine needle aspiration)—Procedure in which a thin needle is inserted into a lesion under ultrasound guidance and moved around to break up the tissue somewhat. Suction is used to pull cells and/or fluid into a syringe for collection. Because there is a 9% rate of false-negative findings or retrieval of an insufficient amount of tissue (no diagnostic), FNA is used less frequently than core biopsy, although it is appropriate to use with lymph nodes or lesions near vascular structures. The procedure is user dependent (i.e., its accuracy depends on the experience of the radiologist performing the procedure), and the risks are similar to those of a blood draw.

Core needle biopsy—Core biopsy is the most common type of biopsy; it is performed in breast imaging because of its high yield of tissue and its accuracy. It is useful for laboratory evaluation of palpable and nonpalpable lesions ranging from mildly suspicious findings to obvious cancers. A hollow needle is used to retrieve a specimen that is about the size of a short spaghetti noodle (i.e., a "core" of tissue); this provides a generous amount of tissue for pathology evaluation. The accuracy is similar to that of surgical biopsy (see Chapter 12).

Stereotactically guided—A mammogram is used to guide the biopsy of the breast. The patient is placed prone (on stomach) on a table that has a hole for placement of the breast; a digital mammogram machine is built into the table underneath. Mammogram images are obtained at +15 degree and − 15 degree angles, and the computer uses a "stereotactic" equation to calculate the depth and location of the lesion in the breast. This gives the radiologist the exact location of the lesion for targeting. The newer high resolution stereotactic units are designed to allow the biopsy to be performed with the patient sitting (upright units) or lying on your stomach (prone unit).

Ultrasound-guided—Ultrasound is used to target the lesion; the radiologist can see the lesion and the needle in real time and can visually guide the needle into the targeted lesion. This is the preferred method of biopsy because of its ease and quickness of performance.

MRI-guided—MRI is used to target the lesion. A limited repeat MRI study with contrast must be performed to reproduce the lesion for targeting. A computer calculates the coordinates and depth of the lesion, and the radiologist uses these data to determine where to place the needle. Because of the length of time necessary for the procedure (i.e., patient comfort and ability to remain still), this technique is used when the lesion is visible only (or best) on MRI.

Surgical—Biopsy performed by a surgeon in the operating room; requires anesthesia, skin incision, and removal of a portion of the breast tissue. This is usually a low-risk and well tolerated procedure, although the risks are greater than with needle biopsy. May be necessary as an initial biopsy procedure if problems with the targeted lesion (e.g., too far back) or with the patient (e.g., severe back pain) are not amenable to needle biopsy. Also used if the lesion is palpable and clinically symptomatic and the patient has opted for excision regardless of the findings.

E. Terms About Biopsy Results

Biopsy—The removal and examination of tissue from a living body to make a precise diagnosis. A pathologist interprets the tissue using a microscope and may perform special tests to determine if the lesion is benign or malignant.

Benign—Not malignant. There is a long list of benign findings.

Atypical—A finding that is not a classically benign type but does not meet the pathology criteria to be called cancer. If it is found as a result of needle biopsy, surgical biopsy is then indicated. (See Chapter 12).

Malignant—A cancer, especially one with the potential to cause death. Most often, the cancer started from breast tissue cells (*primary breast cancer*), but occasionally malignant tumors metastasize to the breast from another source, such as lymph (lymphoma), lung, stomach, or ovary.

Radiologic-pathologic correlation—When a core needle biopsy is performed, every effort is made to confirm the accuracy of the biopsy; because this is a sampling procedure, an error such as missing the lesion or obtaining too little representative tissue could invalidate the result. The imaging findings are compared with the results from examination of the tissue to determine whether they are concordant or discordant. Correlation requires a good working relationship between the radiologist and the pathologist; the final determination from the comparison is the responsibility of the radiologist.

Concordant—The pathology diagnosis and the imaging results "fit." The pathology diagnosis explains the radiographic findings, and the findings are consistent with the diagnosis.

Discordant—The pathology diagnosis and the imaging results do not "fit." The pathology diagnosis does not explain the radiographic findings. Usually this means that the finding on the radiology study was more suspicious than the finding on the pathology report, and there is concern for a false negative result. Surgical excision is usually recommended.

F. Terms About Reporting Your Past Surgical History

Excisional biopsy—Surgical removal of a portion of the breast that includes the abnormality or region of interest. Typically refers to removal of a benign lesion (e.g., fibroadenoma).

Lumpectomy—Surgical procedure to remove cancer or other abnormal tissue. Implies that the final pathology result was cancer.

Mastectomy—Excision of the breast.

    Modified radical—Removal of the breast, pectoralis (chest wall) muscles, axillary (armpit) lymph nodes, and the associated skin and subcutaneous tissue in the treatment of breast cancer. These patients do not require annual screening mammography of the mastectomy site, only of the remaining breast.

    Simple—Removal of only the breast tissue and nipple and a small portion of the overlying skin; these patients may still require annual screening mammography.

    Subcutaneous—Excision of the breast tissue so that the breast form may be reconstructed. May be **Skin sparing which preserves the overlying skin only** or **Nipple sparing**, which preserves the overlying skin, nipple, and areola (pigmented area surrounding nipple). These patients may still require annual screening mammography.

G. Terms About the Frequency of Imaging

Baseline—Refers to your first examination, used to document the "usual" appearance of your breast tissue and as a reference point when subsequent films are taken. Changes from the baseline findings may indicate the presence of disease.

Routine—Examinations are performed on a regular basis, such as every 12 months (annual).

Short-interval follow-up—Follow-up with a mammogram or other breast examination in a time frame that is less than 1 year (usually 6 months). A shorter time frame may be recommended depending on the findings. (such as following trauma related findings or infectons) which may require follow up in 1 or 2 months given that these finding may change in a shorter period of time.

Surveillance—Monitoring of a finding with imaging studies over some interval of time in order to evaluate for stability or change. Usually prescribed (instead of biopsy) for lesions that are considered to be probably benign with very low suspicion for malignancy but that are not clearly benign.

H. General Terms About Imaging Findings

Abnormality—Any finding that is believed not to represent normal breast tissue or is not an expected finding for the particular study. May be benign or suspicious.

Lesion—Broadly, any finding that is worth specific mention in a report, usually a mass or nodule. May be benign or concerning for malignancy.

Conspicuity—Refers to a finding that is becoming more obvious (more visually conspicuous); this may be because the finding is actually increasing or because it is being better seen due to improved technique or positioning.

Nodule—A space-occupying lesion that can be seen in two radiologic projections (i.e., from two viewpoints); a three-dimensional lesion. The term is typically used in reference to smaller lesions.

Mass—A space-occupying lesion that can be seen in two different radiologic projections (i.e., from two viewpoints); a three-dimensional lesion. The term is typically used in reference to larger lesions.

I. Terms Useful for Understanding Mammography

Density—An area of "whiteness" that is seen in only one radiologic view; it lacks the dimensionality to be called a mass or nodule.

Lucency—Refers to tissue that is relatively less dense (less white) compared with the surrounding normal tissue; can imply that fat is present within the lesion. Fat in an imaging abnormality is an extremely favorable finding and usually implies a benign etiology. However, given the significant improvements in resolution of many breast imaging examinations the presence of fat is no longer a slam dunk for a benign process. The characteristics of the lesion must be scutinized even with this finding.

Architectural distortion—Alteration of the normal undulating architecture of the breast tissue, characterized by radiating straight lines from a central point. No visible mass is identified, but its presence is implied by the presence of the distortion. May be an associated finding with other abnormalities.

Calcifications—Deposits of calcium in the breast tissue that are visualized as white specks on a mammogram; they are not related to calcium blood levels or taking calcium supplements. Large and coarse calcifications are benign, whereas tiny calcifications with different shapes are most concerning. The distribution of the calcifications (e.g., clustered, linear) provides clues to the radiologist as to their degree of suspicion for cancer.

J. Terms Useful for Understanding Breast Ultrasound

Echogenicity—Refers to the "color" of an ultrasound finding relative to the background tissue; findings are either hypoechoic (darker than background), hyperechoic (whiter than background), or isoechoic (same as background). Most cancers are hypoechoic.

Shadowing—In an ultrasound examination, the density of the breast (i.e., how thickly packed the tissue is) determines how much of the sound wave can penetrate the tissue. Lesions that have a thin consistency, such as a fluid-filled cyst, do not slow down the sound wave very much, so it goes through quickly. However, lesions that are densely packed block the sound wave and do not allow it to go through, which creates the appearance of a shadow and effectively blocks the acquisition of further information. Because cancers are frequently very dense and have shadowing, this is an unfavorable finding; however, normal tissue that is very dense can also cause shadowing.

Homogeneous—The lesion is all one "color"; the elements within the lesion are similar to one another; this is a favorable characteristic and is commonly seen in benign lesions.

Heterogeneous—Different "colors" are present within the lesion, implying that the lesion is complex to some degree. Heterogeneity increases the concern for malignancy.

Cyst—A lesion that contains a collection of fluid (like a water balloon); it is benign.

Solid—A border-forming mass of tissue; not a cyst.

Tumor—A solid mass of tissue with a defined border or capsule; can be benign or malignant. This can be a specific diagnosis such as benign fibroadenoma (the most common tumor diagnosed in the breast).

K. Terms Useful for Understanding Breast MRI

Enhancement—The accumulation of contrast dye in a specific area. Dye is administered intravenously and transported through the veins to the tissues of the breast, areas with a lot of blood flow "enhance" and thus appear white on the image relative to the background structures. Cancers tend to have more vessels than normal tissue because they are needed to feed the tumor and make it grow. Therefore, enhancement is the primary finding of cancer in breast MRI. Because normal tissue and other tumors and conditions can also enhance, the radiologist looks at the type of enhancement, its shape, and other features to determine the degree of suspicion.

Washout—The contrast dye is quickly taken up and also quickly released by the lesion. This is a finding that is characteristic and very suspicious for cancer.

Plateau—The contrast dye is taken up quickly but does not wash out during the time of the examination; that is, it maintains a steady ("plateau") appearance of whiteness. This type of pattern can be seen in cancers and in benign findings; other features are needed to help to determine the degree of suspicion.

Progressive—The contrast dye is taken up slowly and progressively over time. This type of pattern is most characteristic of benign processes but can also be seen in early-stage cancers such as DCIS.

L. Terms About Lesion Location

O'Clock Position—Defines an axis (straight line) extending from the nipple to the outer edge (peripheral aspect) of the breast. The clock position describes the location of a finding based on viewing the breast as a clock face as seen when facing the patient. This location is different depending on which breast you are discussing; for example, the 10 o'clock axis is located in the upper outer aspect of the right breast but in the upper inner aspect of the left breast. The position of the lesion is further defined by measuring the nipple-to-lesion distance along the designated axis (i.e., the tumor was located at the 9 o'clock position, 3 cm from the nipple).

Quadrant—The location of a breast lesion is commonly described by dividing the breast into four quarters (25% wedges) defined by imaginary lines drawn horizontally and vertically from the nipple. In this system, there is an upper outer quadrant (UOQ), an upper inner quadrant (UIQ), a lower outer quadrant (LOQ), and a lower inner quadrant (LIQ) in each breast.

Retroareolar—Located immediately behind or near the nipple.

Axillary tail—The part of the breast tissue that is located in the far upper outer quadrant and extends towards the axilla.

Axillary—Located in the underarm or armpit. Lymph nodes are located there, and it is the first place to which breast cancer travels when it metastasizes; therefore, evaluation of this area provides information about the spread of disease. Rarely, breast cancer can start in the axilla.

FNP (Distance "*from the nipple*")—Also called nipple-to-lesion distance (NLD). The distance is measured along an axis defined by the o'clock position. This measurement is most useful in patients with large breasts, in whom the axis may span 12 cm or more.

M. Terms About the Distribution of Findings

Solitary—One finding; a single lesion.

Focal—Located in a small, defined area.

Clustered—More than one finding is present in a small area of tissue; for calcifications, this usually implies several calcifications within a volume of 1 cubic centimeter.

Grouped—More than one finding is present in the same region of the breast (but not in a tight cluster).

Diffuse—All over; no particular area is different from the rest.

Scattered—Patchy, random distribution of a finding.

Unilateral—In one breast ("one side").

Bilateral—In both breasts ("both sides").

Ipsilateral—In the same breast ("same side").

Contralateral—In the opposite breast ("opposite side").

N. Terms About Conclusions and Recommendations

BIRADS (Breast Imaging Reporting and Data System)—System developed by the American College of Radiology to provide a standardized language of description (lexicon) and a clear, concise method of reporting data on mammographic studies. This enables clear communication between the radiologist and the referring physician and allows for collection and comparison of data.

Category 0—Incomplete evaluation; additional imaging is needed or awaiting prior films. Additional diagnostic studies may be required to gather more information about a finding before a final decision can be made, or prior films or biopsy reports may be needed to compare with those from the current examination.

Category 1—Negative; no evidence of malignancy; routine imaging is recommended.

Category 2—Benign; a finding is observed but is believed to have no likelihood of malignancy; routine imaging is recommended.

Category 3—Probably benign; a finding is noted but is believed to have an extremely low likelihood of malignancy; short-interval follow-up recommended (imaging surveillance).

Category 4—Suspicious; cancer is a possibility; biopsy is recommended.

Category 5—Highly (very) suspicious; cancer is probable; biopsy is recommended.

Category 6—Known cancer.

O. Terms About Breast Tissue Composition

Fatty—Containing 24% or less fibroglandular tissue.

Average—Containing 25% to 50% fibroglandular tissue; sometimes called Scattered.

Heterogeneously (moderately) dense—Containing 51% to 75% fibroglandular tissue.

Extremely (very) dense—Containing more than 75% fibroglandular tissue.

P. Terms About Physical Examination of the Breast

Palpable—A lesion that can be felt by using the hand (i.e., manual examination, either CBE or SBE).

SBE (Self breast examination)—Breast examination performed by the woman herself. It is recommended that women perform SBE every month starting at age 20 years.

CBE (Clinical breast examination)—A breast examination performed by a healthcare provider; routine annual CBE is recommended. CBE should be performed before a screening mammogram to confirm that it is negative (i.e., the patient is truly a screening patient).

Q. Terms About Breast Surgeries for Benign Conditions

Implant—An implantable device consisting of an outer shell (envelope) filled with material such as silicone, saline, or both (double lumen); it is placed to improve the appearance of the breast shape.

Augmentation—Also called Augmentation mammoplasty. Implants are placed to increase the size or appearance of the breast for cosmetic reasons.

Retropectoral—Implant positioned behind the pectoralis (chest wall) muscle.

Pre-pectoral—Implant positioned in front of the pectoralis muscle; also called Subglandular.

Reduction—Also called Reduction mammoplasty. Removal of large amounts of breast tissue to reduce the size of the breasts. It is performed for benign reasons, either for cosmetic reasons or to alleviate debilitating symptoms related to the weight of large breasts. Results in a characteristic architectural distortion pattern on postoperative imaging.

Lift—Also called Mastopexy. Removal of small amounts breast tissue and skin to "uplift" the breast and provide a cosmetically more pleasing form; may be performed in conjunction with implant placement. Results in a pattern of architectural distortion similar to that of reduction surgery on postoperative imaging.

R. Terms About Cancer-Related Breast Surgeries

Lumpectomy—Surgical removal of a cancerous tumor (lump) together with a portion of the surrounding breast tissue. The goal is to remove all of the known cancer, leaving normal tissue at the edges of the sample (negative margins).

Mastectomy—Excision of the breast; see Terms About Your Surgical History.

Reconstruction—Performed after mastectomy to reconstruct a breast-like form for cosmetic reasons.

Implants—Similar to implants for augmentation, but may use devices with a different outer shell, different filler, or different texture because of technical factors related to a mastectomy site.

Flaps—

TRAM (Transverse rectus abdominis myocutaneous) flap—Type of reconstruction that involves transfer of abdominal muscle, fat, and vessels into the chest to make a breast-like form. These patients may still require annual screening mammography. Deep inferior epigastric perforator (DIEP) flap and latissimus flap reconstruction surgeries are now common and result in a similar imaging appearance mammography may be still indicated in these patients.

DIEP (Deep inferior epigastric perforator) flap—Transfer of abdominal fat and skin that is connected to the deep inferior epigastric perforator vessels. The tissue is dissected with vessels intact, and the deep inferior epigastric vessels are dissected through the abdominal rectus muscle leaving the muscle intact; the vessels and tissue are then transferred to the chest, and a microsurgical anastomosis (closure) is performed to the inframammary vessels to reestablish blood supply. The tissue is then shaped into a breast mound, as with a TRAM flap. This procedure is now common and results in a similar imaging appearance. The main benefit of DIEP flap over TRAM flap is that the abdominal rectus muscle is not sacrificed so the risk of abdominal hernia is lower. Mammography may still be indicated in these patients.

Latissimus dorsi muscle flap—A muscle or myocutaneous flap is used to transfer the latissimus dorsi muscle with or without the skin paddle based on the thoracodorsal vascular bundle. The flap is elevated and then rotated to the breast to add soft tissue. The procedure can be performed with or without a breast implant depending on size desired. This procedure is now common and results in a similar imaging appearance. Mammography may be still indicated in these patients.

Expanders—Temporary implants that are used to stretch tissues before permanent implant placement.

S. Terms About Statistics

Negative—The imaging findings are favorable and suggest a benign condition of the breast.

True negative—No cancer was present, and the radiographic study also showed no evidence of cancer.

False negative—Cancer was present, but the radiographic study did not detect it; known as an "under-call."

Positive—The imaging findings are concerning and suggest that cancer is a possibility.

True positive—Cancer was present, and the radiographic study accurately detected it.

False positive—The radiographic study showed a finding that was thought to be cancer, but further investigation proved it to be benign; known as an over-call.

Sensitivity—Is a statistical measure of the performance of a test; also called the true positive rate, it measures the proportion of positives that are correctly identified (in our case the percentage of breast cancers that are correctly identified as cancer). Theoretically for example, if we reviewed 100 MRI studies each with a finding (10 with cancer as the finding); in our theoretical case the MRI deteted 20 findings that were felt to be suspicious; if all 10 of the cancers we among those felt to be suspicous the sensitivity of the examination is 100%. This is true regardless of how many additional areas are identified; no areas of cancer are being missed.

Specificity—Is a statistical measure of the performance of a test; also called the true negative rate; it measures the proportion of negatives that are correctly identified as such (in our case the percentage of benign tumors that were correctly identified as being benign). For example, in our hypothetical review of 100 MRI studies 80 of the 90 benign tumors were correctly identified as benign, not cancer. Thus, the sensitivity is 89%.

T. Terms About Personnel

Radiologist—A medical doctor and physician imaging expert who is trained in the specialty of radiology (medical school and at least 4 years of residency in diagnostic radiology). Radiologists who interpret mammograms must provide documentation of continuing medical education (CME) hours in mammography and must read a minimum number of mammograms per year to maintain eligibility to interpret these studies. The radiologist assists referring doctors in the care of their patients by supervising the performance of imaging procedures and providing expert assessment of the examinations.

Radiologic technologist—A person who is skilled in the technical performance of radiologic studies. Successful completion of training at a radiologic technology school and state licensure are required. Mammography technologists and breast ultrasound technologists are required to undergo additional specific training in their respective fields; they must document evidence of competency (pass a rigorous test on the physics and clinical performance of their craft) and participate in continuing medical education (CME) on an annual basis. Special training is also required for other types of technologists on the breast imaging team, such as those who perform breast MRI or nuclear medicine studies (e.g., PEM).

Breast patient navigator—Certified specialist who works directly with women at all stages of breast care to answer questions about tests and results, explain procedures, correspond with the referring physician, schedule appointments, and connect you to appropriate resources in the community (your new best friend!). The breast health navigator is available as part of the breast imaging team to women at all stages of breast care—from those coming in for a routine screening examination to those diagnosed with cancer. They provide the much-needed link between the radiologist and the patients and referring clinicians they serve.

RADIOLOGY CONSULT

The goal of any physician in communicating to patients is to impart information in a manner that allows patients to fully understand what is being said and then apply that information to their health care decisions. Please be aware that the meanings of the terms in this section are defined according to their practical use in a breast imaging evaluation and may have a different meaning if used in a different context. Asking for clarification when talking to your doctor will greatly assist your understanding of the data.

Breast Health Vocabulary

QUICK REFERENCE, ALPHABETICAL

Abnormality—Any finding that is believed not to represent normal breast tissue or is not an expected finding for the particular study. May be benign or suspicious.

Architectural distortion—Alteration of the normal undulating architecture of the breast tissue, characterized by radiating straight lines from a central point. No visible mass is identified, but its presence is implied by the presence of the distortion. May be an associated finding with other abnormalities.

Aspiration—Removal of fluid or cells through a needle.

Atypical finding—One that is not a classically benign type but does not meet the pathology criteria to be called cancer. If it is found as a result of needle biopsy, surgical biopsy is then indicated. (See Chapter 12).

Augmentation (Augmentation mammoplasty)—Placement of implants to increase the size or appearance of the breast for cosmetic reasons.

Average breast density—Containing 24% to 50% fibroglandular tissue.

Axilla—The underarm or armpit. Lymph nodes are located there, and it is the first place to which breast cancer travels when it metastasizes; therefore, evaluation of this area provides information about the spread of disease. Rarely, breast cancer can start in the axilla.

Axillary tail—The part of the breast tissue that is located in the far upper outer quadrant and extends towards the axilla.

Baseline—Refers to your first examination, used to document the "usual" appearance of your breast tissue and as a reference point when subsequent films are taken. Changes from the baseline findings may indicate the presence of disease.

Benign—Not malignant; showing no evidence of cancer. There are notable findings, but they have imaging characteristics that are favorable and are not believed to be cancer.

Bilateral—On both sides. The presence of cancer in both breasts may represent two different types of breast cancer.

Biopsy—The removal and examination of tissue from a living body to make a precise diagnosis. A pathologist interprets the tissue using a microscope and may perform special tests to determine if the lesion is benign or malignant.

BIRADS (Breast Imaging Reporting and Data System)—System developed by the American College of Radiology to provide a standardized language of description (lexicon) and a clear, concise method of reporting data on mammographic studies. This enables clear communication between the radiologist and the referring physician and allows for collection and comparison of data. Results and recommendations are reported as BIRADS Category 0 through Category 6. BIRADS lexicon is recommended for breast ultrasound and breast MRI as well.

BIRADS Category 0—Incomplete evaluation; additional imaging is needed or awaiting prior films. Additional diagnostic studies may be required to gather more information about a finding before a final decision can be made, or prior films or biopsy reports may be needed to compare with those from the current examination.

BIRADS Category 1—Negative; no evidence of malignancy; routine imaging is recommended.

BIRADS Category 2—Benign; a finding is observed but is believed to have no likelihood of malignancy; routine imaging is recommended.

BIRADS Category 3—Probably benign; a finding is noted but is believed to have an extremely low likelihood of malignancy; short-interval follow-up is recommended.

BIRADS Category 4—Suspicious; cancer is a possibility; biopsy is recommended.

BIRADS Category 5—Highly suspicious; cancer is probable; biopsy is recommended.

BIRADS Category 6—Known cancer.

Breast patient navigator—Certified specialist who works directly with women at all stages of breast care to answer questions about tests and results, explain procedures, provide cancer education, correspond with the referring physician, and connect patients with appropriate resources in the community (your new best friend!).

BSGI (Breast-specific gamma imaging)—A molecular imaging test in which a radioactive tracer is injected into the patient; the radioactive material preferentially accumulates in tumors (both cancers and some noncancer tumors), and a special gamma camera is used to detect the "activity" in the tumor cells and produce an image.

CAD (Computer-aided detection)—A type of computer software program that can be applied to either film-screen or digital mammogram images. The program scans the film to detect and mark certain suspicious findings, thus alerting the radiologist to examine the area closely. CAD is most useful for detecting small clusters of calcifications that may be missed at first glance.

Calcifications—Deposits of calcium in the breast tissue that are visualized as white specks on a mammogram; they are not related to calcium blood levels or taking calcium supplements. Large and coarse calcifications are benign, whereas tiny calcifications with different shapes are most concerning. The distribution of the calcifications (e.g., clustered, linear) provides clues to the radiologist as to their degree of suspicion for cancer.

Callback—See Recall.

Carcinoma—A malignant new growth made up of breast cells tending to infiltrate the surrounding tissues and give rise to metastases. (See Malignancy.)

Category 0 through Category 6—See BIRADS Category 0 through 6.

CBE (Clinical breast examination)—A breast examination performed by the patient's primary care provider; routine annual CBE is recommended. CBE should be performed before a screening mammogram to confirm that there are no obvious problems.

Clustered findings—More than one finding in a small area of tissue; for calcifications, this usually implies several calcifications within a volume of 1 cubic centimeter.

Computed tomography—See CT.

Computer-aided detection—See CAD.

Concordant—Term used when the pathology diagnosis and the imaging results "fit." The pathology diagnosis explains the radiographic findings, and the findings are consistent with the diagnosis.

Conspicuity—Refers to a finding that is becoming more obvious (more visually conspicuous); this may be because the finding is actually increasing or because it is being better seen due to improved technique or positioning.

Contralateral—Refers to the "other" side of the body relative to a known lesion; opposite of ipsilateral. For example, if a patient has a known right breast cancer, a new finding in the left breast would be described as occurring in the contralateral breast.

Core needle biopsy (Core biopsy)—This is the most common type of biopsy; it is performed in breast imaging because of its high yield of tissue and its accuracy. It is useful for evaluation of palpable and nonpalpable lesions ranging from mildly suspicious findings to obvious cancers. A hollow needle is used to retrieve a specimen that is about the size of a short spaghetti noodle (i.e., a "core" of tissue); this provides a generous amount of tissue for pathology evaluation. The accuracy is similar to that of surgical biopsy (see Chapter 12).

CT (Computed tomography)—Imaging modality in which a series of cross-sectional x-ray images are obtained along a body axis; the computer software can also produce a three-dimensional image. Can reveal anatomic details of internal organs that cannot be seen on conventional x-ray films.

Cyst—A lesion that contains a collection of fluid (like a water balloon); it is benign.

Cyst aspiration—A procedure in which very thin needle is inserted into a cyst (or focal fluid pocket) and the fluid is pulled back into a syringe. In breast imaging, this is done under ultrasound guidance to direct the needle into the cyst and to confirm that all of the fluid has been removed. The risk is similar to that of a blood draw.

DCIS (Ductal carcinoma in situ)—Earliest form of breast cancer; the cancer is fully contained within the straw-shaped breast duct and theoretically has had no chance to spread elsewhere in the body. Likely curable if treated appropriately. Compare IDC.

Density—An area of "whiteness" that is seen in only in one radiologic view; it lacks the dimensionality to be called a mass or nodule.

Diagnosis—Identification of the nature of an illness or other problem by examination of the symptoms and test results.

Diffuse—All over; no particular area is different from the rest.

Digital techniques—Images are acquired and displayed using computer-based technology; this allows for manipulation of the images by the radiologist, which may result in better interpretations and fewer recalls. Found by a large, multisite study to have an advantage over film-screen images in younger women and in women with dense breasts. Currently the standard of care in most facilities.

Discordant—Term used when the pathology diagnosis and the imaging results do not "fit." The pathology diagnosis does not explain the radiographic findings. Usually this means that the finding on the radiology study was more suspicious than the finding on the pathology report, and there is concern for a false-negative result. Surgical excision is usually recommended.

Disposition—The plan of action that is being recommended.

Ductal cancer—See DCIS and IDC.

Echogenicity—Refers to the "color" of an ultrasound finding relative to the background tissue; findings are either hypoechoic (darker than background), hyperechoic (whiter than background), or isoechoic (same as background). Most cancers are hypoechoic.

Enhancement—The accumulation of contrast dye in a specific area in the breast. Dye is administered intravenously and transported through the veins to the tissues of the breast, and areas with a lot of blood flow "enhance" and thus appear white on the MRI image relative to the background tissue. Cancers tend to have more vessels than normal tissue because they are needed to feed the tumor and make it grow. Therefore, enhancement is the primary finding of cancer in breast tissue. Because normal tissue and other tumors and conditions can also enhance, the radiologist looks at the type of enhancement, its shape, and other features to determine the degree of suspicion. Contrast enhanced mammography is a modality that is currently being investigated. It may provide an easier and less costly alternative to MRI. However, to do that it would need to be as good or better than MRI, a mighty tough task given the high sensitivity of MRI.

Excisional biopsy—Surgical removal of a portion of the breast that includes the abnormality or region of interest. The term typically refers to removal of a benign lesion (e.g., fibroadenoma).

Extremely dense breast—Containing more than 75% fibroglandular tissue.

FNA (Fine needle aspiration)—Procedure in which a thin needle is inserted into a lesion under ultrasound guidance and moved around to break up the tissue somewhat. Suction is used to pull cells and/or fluid into a syringe for collection. Because there is a 9% rate of false-negative findings or retrieval of an insufficient amount of tissue (nondiagnostic), FNA is used less frequently than core biopsy, although it is appropriate to use with lymph nodes or lesions near vascular structures. The procedure is user dependent (i.e., its accuracy depends on the experience of the radiologist performing the procedure), and the risks are similar to those of a blood draw.

FNP—Distance of the finding "from the nipple". See Nipple-to-lesion distance.

False negative—Cancer was present, but the radiographic study did not detect it; known as an under-call.

False positive—The radiographic study showed a finding that was thought to be cancer, but further investigation proved it to be benign; known as an over-call.

Fatty breast density—Containing 24% or less fibroglandular tissue.

Film-screen image—Traditional method of acquiring mammogram films. A cassette containing a piece of film captures the image; the film is then run through a processor and developed (as in darkroom photography). The resulting image is evaluated by the radiologist.

Focal finding—Located in a small, defined area.

Grouped findings—More than one finding in the same region of the breast (but not in a tight cluster).

Heterogeneous finding—On ultrasound imaging, different "colors" are present within the lesion, implying that the lesion is complex to some degree. Heterogeneity increases the concern for malignancy. (See Echogenicity.)

Heterogeneously dense breast — Containing 51% to 75% fibroglandular tissue; also called Moderately dense.

Highly suspicious (very suspicious) finding—There is a high probability that the finding is cancer. The finding has the features of cancer, and biopsy is recommended to confirm. There are a few benign conditions (e.g., granular cell tumor) that can also have malignant features and simulate cancer on imaging.

Homogeneous finding—On ultrasound imaging, the lesion is all one "color"; the elements within the lesion are similar to one another; this is a favorable characteristic and is commonly seen in benign lesions. (See Echogenicity.)

IDC (Invasive ductal carcinoma)—The most common type of breast cancer. It arises from the ductal elements in the breast tissue. The pathologist can determine the type by review of the tissue under the microscope and by performing special tests and stains in the laboratory. Compare DCIS.

ILC (Invasive lobular carcinoma)—The second broad group of invasive cancer encountered, but less common than IDC. This type of cancer is difficult to diagnose clinically and also notoriously hard to detect on mammography because its growth pattern is vague and it may not form a mass; it may manifest as subtle changes in density (whiteness) on a mammogram or merely as decreasing size of the breast.

Implants—A breast implant consists of an outer shell (envelope) filled with material such as silicone, saline, or both (double lumen). The device is placed to improve the appearance of the breast shape, either for augmentation or after a breast cancer surgery (lumpectomy or mastectomy).

Invasive cancer—Any breast cancer that has broken through the straw-shaped breast duct or is infiltrating (invading) into the surrounding tissues. These cancers theoretically may have invaded adjacent blood vessels or lymphatic vessels, so metastatic disease is a possibility; the statistical likelihood of metastatic disease can be estimated based on factors including tumor size and grade. See IDC and ILC.

Ipsilateral—Refers to the "same" side of the body relative to a known lesion; opposite of contralateral. For example, if a patient has a known right breast cancer, a new finding in the right breast would be described as occurring in the ipsilateral breast.

Lesion—A broad term used by radiologists to denote a finding that is worth specific mention in a report; usually included in discussions about masses or nodules. May be benign or concerning for malignancy.

Lift (Mastopexy)—Removal of small amounts of breast tissue and skin to "uplift" the breast and provide a cosmetically more pleasing form; may be performed in conjunction with implant placement. Results in a pattern of architectural distortion similar to that of reduction surgery.

Lobular cancer—See ILC.

Lucency—Refers to tissue that is relatively less dense (less white) compared with the surrounding normal tissue; can imply that fat is present within the lesion. Fat in an imaging abnormality is an extremely favorable finding and usually, but not always, implies a benign etiology—this is one of the few times in life when fat is good!

Lumpectomy—Surgical removal of a cancerous tumor (lump) together with a portion of the surrounding breast tissue. The goal is to remove all of the known cancer, leaving normal tissue at the edges of the sample (negative margins).

Magnetic resonance imaging—see MRI.

Malignancy—A broad category of disease that includes carcinomas and other processes; a cancer, especially one with the potential to cause death. In the breast, the most frequently encountered type of malignancy is a carcinoma that started from breast tissue cells (i.e., primary breast cancer), but occasionally a malignant tumor represents a metastasis to the breast from another source such as lymph nodes (lymphoma), lung, stomach, or ovary.

Mammography—Imaging modality in which x-rays are sent through the breast tissue to produce a flat (two-dimensional) representation of the breast. In this image, fatty areas appear gray, and dense areas appear white. Compression of the breast is necessary for acceptable image quality. The associated dose of radiation is very low.

Mass—A space-occupying lesion that can be seen in two different radiologic projections (i.e., from two viewpoints); a three-dimensional lesion. The term is typically used in reference to larger lesions (compare Nodule).

Mastectomy—Excision of the breast; different types include Simple, Modified radical, or Skin-sparing. See "Topics in Breast Imaging: Terms About Your Surgical History."

Metastasis—Spread of cancer in the breast to lymph nodes or other organs or to the opposite breast via blood vessels or lymphatics. Breast cancer spreading outside the confines of the breast is called metastatic breast cancer. This is what accounts for mortality associated with the disease.

Mildly suspicious finding—The possibility of cancer is low, but the finding is concerning enough to warrant biopsy. The benefit of finding a small cancer (one that is likely to be in an early stage and may be curable) is greater than the risk of the procedure. The outcome is statistically more likely to be benign than cancer.

Moderately suspicious finding—The likelihood that the lesion is cancer is approximately as great as the likelihood that it is benign. The finding has features of both benign and malignant conditions; biopsy is warranted for further evaluation.

Modified radical mastectomy—Removal of the breast, pectoralis (chest wall) muscles, axillary (armpit) lymph nodes, and the associated skin and subcutaneous tissue in the treatment of breast cancer. These patients do not require annual screening mammography of the mastectomy site, only of the remaining breast.

Mortality—Death directly related to a particular disease. In the case of breast cancer, the mortality rate varies based on tumor size, tumor grade, distant metastasis, and type of treatment (i.e., surgery, chemotherapy, radiation therapy).

MQSA (Mammography Quality Standards Act of 1992)—Established standards for reporting of findings in mammography and, increasingly, other breast imaging modalities. See BIRADS Category 0 through BIRADS Category 6.

MRI (Magnetic resonance imaging)—Modality that uses extremely strong magnets to cause changes in the tissue (not harmful) so that images can be produced; for breast tissue evaluation, contrast dye containing gadolinium is injected. The way in which the tissue responds to the magnets, the timing of the images, and the amount of dye enhancement provide information about the makeup of the tissue that can be useful in detecting cancers. MRI can be used as an adjunct ("helper") modality along with to standard imaging (mammography and ultrasound) or as a screening tool in high-risk patients.

MRI-guided biopsy—Biopsy in which MRI is used to target the lesion. A limited repeat MRI study with contrast must be performed to reproduce the lesion for targeting. A computer calculates the coordinates and depth of the lesion, and the radiologist uses these data to determine where to place the needle. Because of the length of time necessary for the procedure (i.e., patient comfort and ability to remain still), this technique is used when the lesion is visible only (or best) on MRI.

Multicentric finding—More than one cancer is present, but they are separated from one another by some distance and are in different portions of the breast (i.e., not in the same quadrant of the breast). Lumpectomy may not be possible, and mastectomy may be required.

Multifocal finding—More than one cancer (from the same process) is present, yet they are either adjacent to one another or near one another and are still contained within a 25% wedge (quadrant) of the breast. Lumpectomy is possible based on imaging; other clinical factors need to be considered as well.

Needle biopsy—see Core needle biopsy.

Negative result—No abnormalities were identified; there is no evidence of cancer, based on certain imaging criteria and the ability of that particular examination to detect the finding. The degree of accuracy for detecting breast cancer is different depending on the examination; for example, a negative screening mammogram has a much higher degree of certainty than a negative screening breast ultrasound study when assessing for breast cancer.

Nipple-to-lesion distance—Distance of a focal breast lesion from the nipple; may be indicated as NLD, FN, or FNP ("from the nipple"). The distance is measured along an axis defined by the o'clock position. This measurement is most useful in patients with large breasts, in whom the axis may span 12 cm or more.

Nipple sparing mastectomy - See Subcutaneous mastectomy.

Nodule—A space-occupying lesion that can be seen in two radiologic projections (i.e., from two viewpoints); a three-dimensional lesion. The term is typically used in reference to smaller lesions (compare Mass).

O'Clock position—Defines an axis (straight line) extending from the nipple to the outer edge (peripheral aspect) of the breast. The clock position locates the direction of the axis based on viewing the breast as a clock face as seen when facing the patient. This direction is different depending on which breast you are discussing; for example, the 10 o'clock axis points to the upper outer aspect of the right breast but the upper inner aspect of the left breast. The position of the lesion is further defined by measuring the nipple-to-lesion distance along the designated axis.

Palpable—Refers to a lesion that can be felt by using the hand (i.e., manual examination, either CBE or SBE).

Pathologist—Specialized doctor who examines samples of body tissue in the laboratory for diagnostic purposes.

PEM (Positron emission mammography)—A molecular imaging examination in which uptake of a glucose (sugar)-based tracer chemical is used to detect activity in cancer cells. Cancer activity can be identified before it is visually detectable as a structure or mass.

Percutaneous—Means "through the skin"; refers to biopsies performed with a needle, which requires a puncture through the skin into the breast.

Plateau—A pattern seen in breast MRI. The enhancement dye is taken up quickly but does not wash out during the time of the examination; that is, it maintains a steady ("plateau") appearance of whiteness. This type of pattern can be seen in cancers and in benign findings; other features are needed to help to determine the degree of suspicion.

Positive result—The diagnosis of breast cancer has been confirmed.

Pre-pectoral—Positioning of a breast implant in front of the pectoralis muscle; also called Subglandular positioning.

Probably benign—Very likely to be benign; there is an extremely low likelihood of malignancy. In the assessment of a mammographic finding, it implies a greater than 98% probability that the finding is benign and that biopsy can be safely deferred with appropriate follow-up (surveillance).

Prognosis—The likely course or outcome of a disease or condition.

Progressive enhancement—A pattern seen in breast MRI. The enhancement dye is taken up slowly and progressively over time. This type of pattern is most characteristic of benign processes but can also be seen in early-stage cancers such as DCIS.

Quadrant—The location of a breast lesion is commonly described by dividing the breast into four quarters (25% wedges) defined by imaginary lines drawn horizontally and vertically from the nipple. In this system, there is an upper outer quadrant (UOQ), an upper inner quadrant (UIQ), a lower outer quadrant (LOQ), and a lower inner quadrant (LIQ) in each breast.

Radiography—Production of an image on a sensitive plate or film by x-rays, gamma rays, or similar radiation.

Radiologic technologist—A person who is skilled in the technical performance of radiologic studies. Successful completion of training at a radiologic technology school and state licensure are required. Mammography technologists and breast ultrasound technologists are required to undergo additional specific training in their respective fields; they must document evidence of competency (pass a rigorous test on the physics and clinical performance of their craft) and participate in continuing medical education (CME) on an annual basis. Special training is also required for other types of technologists on the breast imaging team, such as those who perform breast MRI or nuclear medicine studies (e.g., PEM).

Radiologic-pathologic correlation—When a core needle biopsy is performed, every effort is made to confirm the accuracy of the biopsy; because this is a sampling procedure, an error such as missing the lesion or obtaining too little representative tissue could invalidate the result. The imaging findings are compared with the results from examination of the tissue to determine whether they are concordant or discordant. Correlation requires a good working relationship between the radiologist and the pathologist; the final determination from the comparison is the responsibility of the radiologist.

Radiologist—A medical doctor who is trained in the specialty of radiology (medical school and at least 4 years of residency in diagnostic radiology). Radiologists who interpret mammograms must provide documentation of continuing medical education (CME) hours in mammography and must read a minimum number of mammograms per year to maintain eligibility to interpret these studies. The radiologist assists referring doctors in the care of their patients by supervising the performance of imaging procedures and providing expert interpretation of the examinations.

Recall—Occurs when you have had a screening mammogram and are requested to return for additional imaging because the radiologist needs further clarification before making a final recommendation.

Reconstruction—A surgical procedure that is performed after mastectomy to reconstruct a breast-like form for cosmetic reasons.

Reduction (Reduction mammoplasty)—Removal of large amounts of breast tissue to reduce the size of the breasts. It is performed for benign reasons, either for cosmetic reasons or to alleviate debilitating symptoms related to the weight of large breasts. Results in a characteristic architectural distortion pattern on imaging.

Retroareolar—Located immediately behind or near the nipple.

Retropectoral—Positioning of a breast implant behind the pectoralis (chest wall) muscle.

Routine imaging—Examinations are performed on a regular basis, such as every year (annual).

SBE (Self breast examination)—Breast examination performed by the woman herself. It is recommended that women perform SBE every month starting at age 20 years.

Scattered—Patchy, random distribution of a finding.

Sensitivity—Is a statistical measure of the performance of a test; also called the true positive rate, it measures the proportion of positives that are correctly identified (in our case the percentage of breast cancers that are correctly identified as cancer). Theoretically for example, if we reviewed 100 MRI studies each with a finding (10 with cancer as the finding); in our theoretical case the MRI deteted 20 findings that were felt to be suspicious; if all 10 of the cancers we among those felt to be suspicous the sensitivity of the examination is 100%. This is true regardless of how many additional areas are identified; no areas of cancer are being missed. Compare Specificity.

Shadowing—In an ultrasound examination, the density of the breast (i.e., how thickly packed the tissue is) determines how much of the sound wave can penetrate the tissue. Lesions that have a thin consistency, such as a fluid-filled cyst, do not slow down the sound wave very much, so it goes through quickly. However, lesions that are densely packed block the sound wave and do not allow it to go through, which creates the appearance of a shadow and effectively blocks the acquisition of further information. Because cancers are frequently very dense and have shadowing, this is an unfavorable finding; however, normal tissue that is very dense can also cause shadowing.

Short-interval follow-up—Follow-up with a mammogram or other breast examination in less than 1 year (usually 6 months). This may be recommended in a shorter interval of time depending on the findings (ie trauma related findings and infection which may change quickly).

Simple mastectomy—Excision of only the breast tissue and nipple and a small portion of the overlying skin; these patients may still require annual screening mammography.

Skin-sparing mastectomy—See Subcutaneous mastectomy.

Solid lesion—A border-forming mass of tissue; not a cyst.

Solitary finding—One finding; a single lesion.

Specificity—Is a statistical measure of the performance of a test; also called the true negative rate; it measures the proportion of negatives that are correctly identified as such (in our case the percentage of benign tumors that were correctly identified as being benign For example, in our hypothetical review of 100 MRI studies 80 of the 90 benign tumors were correctly identified as benign, not cancer. Thus, the sensitivity is 89%, Compare Sensitivity.

Stereotactically guided (mammogram-guided) biopsy—A mammogram is used to guide the biopsy of the breast. The patient is placed prone (on stomach) on a table that has a hole for placement of the breast; a digital mammogram machine is built into the table underneath. Mammogram images are obtained at +15 degree and -15 degree angles, and the computer uses a "stereotactic" equation to calculate the depth and location of the lesion in the breast. This gives the radiologist the exact location of the lesion for targeting. Newer higher resolution upright units are becoming popular as well.

Subcutaneous mastectomy -Excision of the breast tissue with preservation of the overlying skin (skin sparing) or with the preservation of the overlying skin, nipple, and areola (nipple sparing) so that the breast form may be reconstructed; these patients may still require annual screening mammography.

Surgical biopsy—Biopsy performed by a surgeon in the operating room; requires anesthesia, skin incision, and removal of a portion of the breast tissue. This is usually a low-risk and well tolerated procedure, although the risks are greater than with needle biopsy. May be necessary as an initial biopsy procedure if problems with the targeted lesion (e.g., too far back) or with the patient (e.g., severe back pain) are not amenable to needle biopsy. Also used if the lesion is palpable and clinically symptomatic and the patient has opted for excision regardless of the findings.

Surveillance—Monitoring of a finding with imaging studies over some interval of time in order to evaluate for stability or change. Usually recommended (instead of biopsy) for lesions that are considered to be probably benign with very low suspicion for malignancy but that are not clearly benign.

Suspicious finding—The finding is concerning for malignancy; the degree of the concern can vary. Biopsy is recommended for suspicious findings so that tissue can be obtained and sent to the laboratory for confirmation. The concern for cancer may be termed mildly, moderately, or very suspicious.

Synchronous—The simultaneous occurrence of two events; in regard to breast cancer, two or more cancers are diagnosed in one or both breasts at or about the same time. They may represent two different types of cancer (e.g., one may be an IDC, and the other may be an ILC).

TRAM (Transverse rectus abdominis myocutaneous reconstruction)—Transfer of abdominal muscle, fat, and vessels into the chest to make a breast-like form (also called a TRAM flap). These patients may still require annual screening mammography.

Tomosynthesis (3-D mammography or tomography)—Imaging modality in which multiple, thin-slice mammographic images are acquired, allowing the radiologist to see inside the depths of the breast, similar to a CT examination. Instead of two images per breast, there may be 150 to 200 images, providing a considerable amount of additional information and a higher confidence level for reporting a study as benign. As the "optimal" mammogram, this modality is useful for all breast densities, but especially in women with dense breasts. In the screening population, 3-D mammography offers at least a 30% decrease in recalls. Lesions that are real are seen better, and some are seen only on the tomographic images, leading to increased detection of small invasive cancers, which is the goal. As the person who interprets the examination, I can say that if I were queen, everyone would have a 3-D screening mammogram!

True negative—No cancer was present, and the radiographic study also showed no evidence of cancer.

True positive—Cancer was present, and the radiographic study accurately detected it.

Tumor—A solid mass of tissue with a defined border or capsule; can be benign or malignant. This can be a specific diagnosis such as benign fibroadenoma (the most common tumor diagnosed in the breast).

Ultrasound (sonography)—Imaging modality that uses sound waves to generate an image. An ultrasound technologist (or the radiologist) puts a probe on the skin and can see inside to the tissue. It is primarily used to determine whether a lesion is a cyst (fluid) or solid (tumor). Commonly used as an adjunct ("helper") technique to better characterize a mammographic finding or to assess for palpable lesions. Ultrasound increasingly plays a role as an supplemental screening examination (in addition to screening mammography), especially in women with dense breast tissue.

Ultrasound-guided biopsy—Ultrasound is used to target the lesion; the radiologist can see the lesion and the needle in real time and can visually guide the needle into the targeted lesion. This is the preferred method of biopsy because of its ease and quickness of performance.

Unilateral—On one side only; cancer is present in one breast (either left or right), but not in both.

Washout—A pattern seen in breast MRI. The enhancement dye is quickly taken up and also quickly released by the lesion. This is a finding that is characteristic and very suspicious for cancer.

Bibliography

CHAPTER I

Berg WA, Zhang Z, Lehrer D, et al. Detection of breast cancer with addition of annual screening ultrasound or a single screening MRI to mammography in women with elevated breast cancer risk. *JAMA*. 2012;307(13):1394–1404.

Centers for Disease Control and Prevention. Breast cancer statistics. https://www.cdc.gov/cancer/breast/statistics. Accessed February 8, 2017.

Eklund GW, Busby RC, Miller SH, Job JS. Improved imaging of the augmented breast. *AJR Am J Roentgenol*. 1988;151(3):469–473.

Kopans DB. *Breast Imaging*. 3rd ed. Philadelphia: Lippincott Williams & Wilkins; 2006.

Lee CH, Dershaw DD, Kopans D, et al. Breast cancer screening with imaging: recommendations from the Society of Breast Imaging and the ACR on the use of mammography, breast MRI, breast ultrasound, and other technologies for the detection of clinically occult breast cancer. *J Am Coll Radiol*. 2010;7(1):18–27.

Morris EA, Schwartz LH, Dershaw DD, van Zee KJ, Abramson AF, Liberman L. MR imaging of the breast in patients with occult primary breast carcinoma. *Radiology*. 1997;205(2):437–440.

Parker SH, Lovin JD, Jobe WE, Burke BJ, Hopper KD, Yakes WF. Nonpalpable breast lesions: stereotactic automated large-core biopsies. *Radiology*. 1991;180(2):403–407.

Pisano ED, Hendrick RE, Yaffe MJ, et al. Diagnostic accuracy of digital versus film mammography: exploratory analysis of selected population subgroups in DMIST. *Radiology*. 2008;246(2):376–383.

Rose SL, Tidwell AL, Bujnoch LJ, Kushwaha AC, Nordmann AS, Sexton R Jr. Implementation of breast tomosynthesis in a routine screening practice: an observational study. *AJR Am J Roentgenol.* 2013;200(6):1401–1408.

Stavros AT. *Breast Ultrasound.* Philadelphia: Lippincott William & Wilkins; 2004.

Tabár L, Vitak B, Chen HH, Yen MF, Duffy SW, Smith RA. Beyond randomized controlled trials: organized mammographic screening substantially reduces breast carcinoma mortality. *Cancer.* 2001;91(9):1724–1731.

Sickles EA. Management of probably benign breast lesions. *Radiol Clin North Am.* 1995;33(6):1123–1130.

CHAPTER 2

American College of Radiology (ACR), Society of Breast Imaging (SBI) joint statement on USPSTF recommendations. https://www.acr.org/Quality-Safety/Resources/Breast-Imaging-Resources. Accessed February 8, 2017.

Andersson I, Janzon L. Reduced breast cancer mortality in women under age 50: updated results from the Malmö Mammographic Screening Program. *J Natl Cancer Inst Monogr.* 1997;22:63–67.

Bernardi D, Macaskill P, Pellegrini M, Valentini M, et al. Breast cancer screening with tomo-synthesis (3D mammography) with acquired or synthetic 2D mammography compared with 2D mammography alone (STORM-2): a population-based prospective study. *Lancet Oncol.* 2016;17(8):1105–1113.

Bjurstam N, Björneld L, Duffy SW, et al. The Gothenburg breast screening trial: first results on mortality, incidence, and mode of detection for women ages 39–49 years at randomization. *Cancer.* 1997;80(11):2091–2099.

Chu KC, Smart CR, Tarone RE. Analysis of breast cancer mortality and stage distribution by age for the Health Insurance Plan clinical trial. *J Natl Cancer Inst.* 1988;80(14):1125–1132.

Ciatto S, Houssami N, Bernardi D, et al. Integration of 3D digital mammography with tomo-synthesis for population breast-cancer screening (STORM): a prospective comparison study. *Lancet Oncol.* 2013;14(7):583–589.

Duffy SW, Agbaje O, Tabar L, et al. Overdiagnosis and overtreatment of breast cancer: estimates of overdiagnosis from two trials of mammographic screening for breast cancer. *Breast Cancer Res.* 2005;7(6):258–265.

Feig SA. Number needed to screen: appropriate use of this new basis for screening mammography guidelines. *AJR Am J Roentgenol.* 2012;198(5):1214–1217.

Feig SA. Pitfalls in accurate estimation of overdiagnosis: implications for screening policy and compliance. *Breast Cancer Res.* 2013;15(4):105.

Friedewald SM, Rafferty EA, Rose SL, et al. Breast cancer screening using tomosynthesis in com-bination with Digital Mammography. *JAMA.* 2014;311(24):2499–2507.

Miller AB, Wall C, Baines CJ, Sun P, To T, Narod SA. Twenty-five year follow-up for breast can-cer incidence and mortality of the Canadian National Breast Screening Study: randomised screening trial. *BMJ.* 2014;348:g366.

Nyström L, Bjurstam N, Jonsson H, Zackrisson S, Frisell J. Reduced breast cancer mortality after 20+ years of follow-up in the Swedish randomized controlled mammography trials in Malmö, Stockholm, and Göteborg. *J Med Screen.* 2016;pii:0969141316648987 [Epub ahead of print].

Nyström L, Larsson LG, Wall S, et al. An overview of the Swedish randomised mammography trials: total mortality pattern and the representivity of the study cohorts. *J Med Screen.* 1996;3(2):85–87.

Rose SL, Tidwell AL, Bujnoch LJ, Kushwaha AC, Nordmann AS, Sexton R Jr. Implementation of breast tomosynthesis in a routine screening practice: an observational study. *AJR Am J Roentgenol.* 2013;200:1401–1408.

Shapiro S. Periodic screening for breast cancer: the HIP Randomized Controlled Trial. Health Insurance Plan. *J Natl Cancer Inst Monogr.* 1997;(22):27–30.

Skaane P, Bandos AI, Gullien R, et al. Comparison of digital mammography alone and digital mammography plus tomosynthesis in a population-based screening program. *Radiology.* 2013;267(1):47–56.

Tabár L, Fagerberg G, Duffy SW, Day NE. The Swedish two county trial of mammographic screening for breast cancer: recent results and calculation of benefit. *J Epidemiol Community Health.* 1989;43(2):107–114.

Tabár L, Tony Chen HH, Amy Yen MF, et al. Mammographic tumor features can predict long-term outcomes reliably in women with 1–14-mm invasive breast carcinoma., *Cancer.* 200415;101(8):1745–1759.

Tabár L, Vitak B, Chen TH, et al. Swedish two-county trial: impact of mammographic screening on breast cancer mortality during 3 decades. *Radiology.* 2011;260(3):658–663.

Tabár L, Vitak B, Chen HH, Yen MF, Duffy SW, Smith RA. Beyond randomized controlled trials: organized mammographic screening substantially reduces breast carcinoma mortality. *Cancer.* 2001;91(9):1724–1731.

CHAPTER 4

American Society of Radiologic Technologists (ASRT). News and announcements. https://www.asrt.org. Accessed February 9, 2017.

CHAPTER 5

Mammography Quality Standards Reauthorization Act of 1998. Public Law 105-248. 42 USC §263b. http://www.gpo.gov/fdsys/pkg/PLAW-105publ248/html/PLAW-105publ248.htm. Accessed February 9, 2017.

Monsees BS. The Mammography Quality Standards Act: an overview of the regulations and guidance. *Radiol Clin North Am.* 2000;38:759–772.

CHAPTER 8

Kopans DB. *Breast Imaging.* 3rd ed. Philadelphia: Lippincott Williams & Wilkins; 2006.

CHAPTER 9

American College of Radiology Appropriateness criteria for breast cancer screening. https://acsearch.acr.org/docs/70910/Narrative/. Accessed February 10, 2017.

Kopans DB. *Breast Imaging.* 3rd ed. Philadelphia: Lippincott Williams & Wilkins; 2006.

CHAPTER 10

American College of Radiology. Appropriateness criteria for breast pain. https://www.guide-lines.gov/summaries/summary/50422/acr-appropriateness-criteria--breast-pain. Accessed February 11, 2017.

American College of Radiology. Appropriateness criteria for nonpalpable mammographic findings (excluding calcifications). https://acsearch.acr.org/docs/69494/Narrative/. Accessed February 11, 2017.

American College of Radiology. Appropriateness criteria for palpable breast masses. https://acsearch.acr.org/docs/69495/Narrative/. Accessed February 11, 2017.

American College of Radiology. *ACR BI-RADS Atlas: Breast Imaging Reporting and Data System.* 5th ed. Reston, VA: American College of Radiology; 2013.

Kopans DB. *Breast Imaging.* 3rd ed. Philadelphia: Lippincott Williams & Wilkins; 2006.

Korn M. Unexpected focal hyper metabolic activity in the breast: significance in patients undergoing 18F-FDG PET/CT. *American Journal of Roentgenology.* 2006 July;187(1):81–85.

CHAPTER 11

Kopans DB. *Breast Imaging.* 3rd ed. Philadelphia: Lippincott Williams & Wilkins; 2006.

CHAPTER 13

Kopans DB. *Breast Imaging.* 3rd ed. Philadelphia: Lippincott Williams & Wilkins; 2006.

CHAPTER 14

American College of Radiology. Appropriateness criteria for stage 1 breast cancer: initial workup and surveillance for local recurrence and distant metastases in asymptomatic women. https://acsearch.acr.org/docs/69496/Narrative/. Accessed February 13, 2017.

Kopans DB. *Breast Imaging.* 3rd ed. Philadelphia: Lippincott Williams & Wilkins; 2006.

CHAPTER 15

Kopans DB. *Breast Imaging.* 3rd ed. Philadelphia: Lippincott Williams & Wilkins; 2006.

CHAPTER 18

Kopans DB. Mammography screening is saving thousands of lives, but will it survive medical malpractice? *Radiology.* 2004;230(1):20–24.

CHAPTER 19

American College of Radiology. ACR practice guideline for imaging pregnant or potentially pregnant adolescents and women with ionizing radiation. https://www.acr.org/~/media/ACR/Documents/PGTS/guidelines/Pregnant_Patients.pdf. Accessed February 15, 2017.

Hendrick RE. Radiation Dose in Women's Imaging: Are we scared yet? *Radiology.* 2010;257(1):246–253.

CHAPTER 20

American College of Radiology. *ACR BI-RADS Atlas: Breast Imaging Reporting and Data System.* 5th ed. Reston, VA: American College of Radiology; 2013.

American College of Radiology. ACR statement on reporting breast density in mammography: reports and patient summaries. Available at http://bit.ly/OXte9y. Accessed February 21, 2017.

Dense breast tissue and screening: *Radiology Today* interview with Carol H. Lee, MD, FACR. *Radiol Today.* 2014;15(1):30.

Index

Note: Page numbers followed by the letters *b* or *f* indicate material found in boxes or figures.

abnormality
  evaluation/diagnoses of, 127
  recall for, 71–72
  term use/definition, 187, 197
abscesses, 111–12, 126
age criteria/guidelines
  in diagnostic evaluation, 67
  for screening mammography, 64–65
agencies, overseeing breast imaging, 36–37
American Cancer Society (ACS), 7, 11, 13,
    38, 176
American College of Obstetrics and Gynecology
    (ACOG), 12, 56, 177
American College of Radiology (ACR), 12, 36,
    56, 151, 169, 191
American Society of Radiologic Technologists
    (ASRT), 34
anatomy, of the breast, 60*f*
anxiety
  decrease of, 163
  of diagnostic patients, 3–6
  diagnostic process and, 39, 66, 71, 110
  imaging surveillance and, 101
  lesion management and, 123

MRI results and, 100
  USPSTF/ACS recommendations and, 11,
    13, 15, 19
Appropriateness Criteria (ACR), 36–37
architectural distortion
  illustration of, 85*f*
  recall/callbacks for, 85–87
  term use/definition, 188, 197
aspiration
  of cysts, 123–26, 124*f*, 184, 199
  FNA, 184–85, 200–1
  term use/definition, 197
asymmetric density. *See also* density/breast
    density
  illustration of, 83*f*
  recall/callbacks for, 82–84
asymptomatic patients, screening of, 57*f*
atypical/atypical finding, term use/definition,
    186, 197
augmentation (augmentation mammoplasty).
    See also implants
  imaging considerations, 152–53
  term use/definition, 192, 197
average, term use/definition, 191

average breast density, term use/definition, 197
axilla, term use/definition, 197
axillary, term use/definition, 190
axillary dissection, architectural distortion
    after, 85
axillary tail, term use/definition, 190, 197

Barnard, Fred R., 43
baseline, term use/definition, 187, 198
BB markers, use of, 89, 90f, 92
benign, term use/definition, 180, 186, 198
benign biopsy, follow-up of, 102–4
benign condition surgeries, terms about, 192
benign evaluation/diagnoses
    bilateral calcifications, 135, 136f
    bilateral nodularity, 135
    of calcifications, 130–32
    of cysts, 129, 129f
    to explain abnormalities, 127
    of fibroadenomas, 128
    fibrocystic changes, 135
    of free silicone, 130
    of hamartomas, 131
    of lipomas, 132
    of lymph nodes, 133
    of sebaceous glands/cysts, 133–34
    of secretory disease, 134
    of skin calcifications, 134
    of skin lesions, 134, 134f
    of trauma areas, 133
    of vascular calcifications, 134–35
Berg, W. A., 7
bilateral, term use/definition, 182, 191, 198
bilateral calcifications, 135, 136f
bilateral nodularity, 135, 137f
biopsy, term use/definition, 186, 188
biopsy results, terms about, 186
BIRADS (Breast Imaging Reporting and Data
    System)
    Category 0 through Category 6,
        69–70, 81
    as quality assurance tool, 37
    term use/definition, 191, 198
BRCA gene mutation, 176
BRCA positivity, 64–65
breast, anatomy of, 60f
breast abscess, 112f. See also abscesses
breast augmentation. See augmentation
    (augmentation mammoplasty)

breast cancer
    follow-up after, 104–7
    incidence of, 5–6
    personal history of, 63
    risk factors for, 18–19
breast density. See also asymmetric density; fatty
        breasts/fatty breast density
    controversy about, 173–78
    HRT and, 82, 103
    screening women with dense breasts, 62
    term use/definition, 188, 197, 200
    types of, 58–59f, 174b
breast examinations. See CBE (clinical
        breast examination); SBE (self breast
        examination)
breastfeeding/lactation, 152
breast health history, knowledge
    of, 26–27
breast imaging
    agencies overseeing, 36–37
    diagnostic evaluation scenarios, 3–5
    patients' understanding of, 9
    as radiology subspecialty, 6–7
    technological advances in, 7–8
    tools/modalities of, 7
    women's advocacy and, 7
Breast Imaging Reporting and Data System
        (BIRADS). See BIRADS (Breast Imaging
        Reporting and Data System)
breast imaging studies/equipment, terms
    about, 183–84
breast imaging tests. See CAD (computer-
        aided detection); mammography;
        molecular imaging; MRI (magnetic
        resonance imaging); tomosynthesis (3-D
        mammography); ultrasound
        (sonography)
breast MRI terms, 189. See also MRI (magnetic
        resonance imaging)
breast patient navigator, term use/definition,
        195, 198
breast-specific gamma imaging. See BSGI
        (breast-specific gamma imaging)
breast tissue composition
    fatty breasts, 130
    terms about, 191
breast ultrasound technologists, 35, 82, 176,
        183, 194, 205, 207. See also radiologic
        technologist (RT)

BSGI (breast-specific gamma imaging)
  as molecular imaging, 48–49
  risk-benefit ratio of, 171
  term use/definition, 184, 198

CAD (computer-aided detection)
  as breast imaging test, 47–48
  reading/interpretation of, 61–62
  term use/definition, 184, 198
calcifications
  benign evaluation/diagnoses of, 132–33
  characteristics of, 77
  illustration of, 16f, 76f
  recall/callbacks for, 74–78
  term use/definition, 188, 199
calcified fibroadenoma, 128f. See also
    fibroadenomas
callback. See recall/callbacks
cancer, terms about, 181–83
cancer-related breast surgeries, terms
    about, 192–93
carcinoma, term use/definition, 181, 199
Category 0 through Category 6. See BIRADS
    (Breast Imaging Reporting and Data
    System)
CBE (clinical breast examination)
  patient questions about, 160
  term use/definition, 192, 199
  USPSTF recommendations for, 12
Centers of Excellence (COE), 36
change in breast size, diagnostic evaluation
    of, 99–100
chest irradiation, personal history of, 63
clinical breast examination. See CBE (clinical
    breast examination)
clustered/clustered findings, term use/definition,
    190, 199
computed tomography (CT). See CT
    (computed tomography)
computer-aided detection. See CAD
    (computer-aided detection)
conclusions and recommendations, terms
    about, 191
concordant, term use/definition, 186
conspicuity, term use/definition, 188
contralateral, term use/definition, 182, 191
contrast mammography, 44
controversial recommendations, for screening
    mammography, 11–13

Cooper's ligaments, 85, 88, 130f
core needle biopsy, term use/definition, 185
CT (computed tomography)
  risk-benefit ratio of, 169–70
  term use/definition, 199
Curie, Marie, 53
current status, knowledge of, 27–28
cyst aspiration
  as image-guided procedure, 123–26, 124f
  term use/definition, 184, 199
cysts
  characteristic appearance of, 80f
  evaluation/diagnoses of, 4, 129, 129f
  patient questions about, 161
  term use/definition, 189, 199
  types of, 129f

Dalai Lama, 127
DCIS (ductal carcinoma in situ)
  illustration of, 16f
  overdiagnosis of, 15
  term use/definition, 181, 200
degenerating fibroadenomas, 128. See also
    fibroadenomas
density/breast density. See also asymmetric
    density; fatty breasts/fatty breast density
  controversy about, 173–78
  HRT and, 82, 103
  screening women with dense breasts, 62
  term use/definition, 188, 197, 200
  types of, 58–59f, 174b
diagnosis, term use/definition, 200
diagnostic evaluation, in recalls/callbacks
  of architectural distortion, 85–87
  of asymmetric density, 82–84
  of calcifications, 74–78
  of well-defined nodules/masses, 78–82
diagnostic evaluation, of history requiring
    special attention
  breast cancer/lumpectomy, 104–7
  incidental findings, 107–9
  previous benign biopsy, 102–4
  previous lesion reported as probably benign,
    100–102
  primary tumor search with metastatic
    disease, 109–10
diagnostic evaluation, of physical findings
  of change in breast size, 99–100
  of nipple discharge, 92–97

diagnostic evaluation, of physical findings (*cont.*)
    of pain/swelling, 91–92
    of palpable abnormality, 89–91
    of skin changes, 97–99
diagnostic evaluation, of symptomatic patients
    age criteria/guidelines, 67
    as anxiety-provoking, 66
    diagnostic symptoms, 68*b*
    indications for, 67–69
    of physical findings, 87–89
    recalls/callbacks, 71–73
    reporting categories, 69–71
diagnostic evaluation scenarios
    of architectural distortion, 86–87
    of asymmetric density, 84
    of calcifications, 77–78
    of changes in breast size, 99–100
    of incidental findings, 107–9
    of nipple discharge, 95–97
    of nodules/masses, 79–82
    of pain/swelling, 91–92
    of palpable abnormality, 89–90
    patient examples, 3–5
    of recall after screening mammogram, 73–74
    of skin changes, 98
diagnostic mammogram. *See also* mammogram;
        mammography; screening mammography
    for asymmetric density, 84
    for calcifications, 77
    in follow-up imaging, 103
    with history of breast cancer, 106
    in imaging surveillance, 100, 102
    for nipple discharge, 96, 97
    patient questions about, 161–62
    for poorly defined nodule/mass, 81
    referral-consult relationship and, 40
    vs. screening mammogram, 10
diagnostic patients, 53, 54*f*
diagnostic study, description of, 53, 55
diagnostic symptoms, 68*b*
DIEP (deep inferior epigastric perforator) flap,
        term use/definition, 193
diffuse, term use/definition, 190, 200
digital/digital techniques, term use/definition,
        183, 200
digital mammography, 7, 18, 44, 171
dimpling, 54*t*, 68*b*, 97. *See also* skin changes
discharge, diagnostic evaluation of
    nipple, 92–97

discordant, term use/definition, 186, 200
disposition, term use/definition, 200
distortion. *See* architectural distortion
distribution of findings, terms about, 190–91
ductal, term use/definition, 182
ductal cancer, term use/definition, 200
ductal carcinoma in situ (DCIS)
    illustration of, 16*f*
    overdiagnosis of, 15
    term use/definition, 181, 200

echogenicity, term use/definition, 188, 200
Ecklund, G. W., 7
emergencies, in breast imaging, 111–33
enhancement, term use/definition, 189, 200
estrogen/estrogen levels, 92–93, 155
excisional biopsy
    appearance on imaging, 26
    architectural distortion after, 85
    postoperative complication evaluation, 113
    term use/definition, 186, 200
expanders, term use/definition, 193
extremely dense breast, term use/definition,
        191, 200

false negative
    as evaluation outcome, 127
    term use/definition, 194, 201
false positive
    breast density and, 177
    as evaluation outcome, 127
    term use/definition, 194, 201
    USPSTF recommendations and, 13
family history
    knowledge of, 25–26, 63
    patient questions about, 160–61
fat necrosis, 133*f*, 146
fatty breasts/fatty breast density
    in benign diagnosis, 130
    image of, 130*f*
    term use/definition, 191, 201
favorable calcifications, 77*f*. *See also* calcifications
federal/state agencies, overseeing breast
        imaging, 36–37
Feig, S. A., 15
fibroadenomas
    as benign diagnoses, 5, 90, 99, 121, 128,
        189, 207
    patient questions about, 161

fibrocystic breast, 88, 159–60

fibrocystic changes, 54*t*, 57*b*, 68*b*, 74, 88, 92, 121, 127, 135, 160

fibrocystic disease, 88, 114

film-screen/film-screen image, 183, 201

film-screen mammography, 44

films/reports retrieval of, 23–25

flaps, term use/definition, 193

fluid drainage/aspiration, 126

FNA (fine needle aspiration), term use/ definition, 184–85, 200–1

FNP (distance "*from the nipp*le"), 190, 201. *See also* nipple-to-lesion distance (NLD)

focal/focal finding, term use/definition, 190, 201

Ford, Henry, 66

free silicone, 27, 130–31, 131*f*

frequency of imaging, terms about, 187

grouped/grouped findings, term use/definition, 190, 201

gynecomastia, 154–55

hamartomas, 131

heterogeneous/heterogeneous finding, term use/definition, 189, 191, 201

highly suspicious finding, term use/definition, 181, 201

high-risk biopsy findings, 64

high-risk populations, 63–64

history
  of breast cancer, 63, 104, 106
  past surgical history terms, 186–87
  patient history knowledge, 25–27

history, requiring special attention
  incidental findings, 107–9
  previous benign biopsy, 102–4
  previous breast cancer/lumpectomy, 104–7
  previous lesions, 100–102
  primary tumor search (metastatic disease), 109–10

homogeneous/homogeneous finding, term use/definition, 189, 201

HRT (hormone replacement therapy)
  breast parenchyma and, 87
  density of breast tissue and, 82, 103
  fibrocystic changes and, 92–93
  side effects of, 79

IDC (invasive ductal carcinoma), term use/definition, 201

ILC (invasive lobular carcinoma)
  asymmetry and, 83
  term use/definition, 182, 201

image-guided procedures
  cyst aspiration, 123–26, 124*f*
  fluid drainage/aspiration, 126
  lesion choice, 114–15
  MRI-guided needle biopsy, 119–20, 119*f*
  radiologic-pathologic correlation, 121–23
  stereotactically guided needle biopsy, 117–19, 117*f*
  ultrasound-guided core biopsy, 115–16, 115*f*

image interpretation, 60–62

imaging findings, terms about, 180–81, 187–88

implants
  appearance on imaging, 27
  architectural distortion after, 85
  free silicone and, 131, 131*f*
  imaging considerations, 152–53
  patient questions about, 161
  postsurgical complication assessment, 112
  term use/definition, 192, 193, 201
  valves manifesting as lumps in, 132*f*

incidental findings, diagnostic evaluation of, 107–9

inflammatory breast cancer, 99, 111–13

interpretation, of mammograms, 60–62

invasive/invasive breast cancer
  asymmetry and, 83
  stages of development, 17*f*
  term use/definition, 181–82, 201–3

ipsilateral, term use/definition, 182, 191, 202

Kopans, D. B., 3, 8, 11

lactation/breastfeeding, 152

Latham, Peter Mere, 111

latissimus dorsi muscle flap, 193

Leifer, Carol, 5

lesion, term use/definition, 187, 202

lesion choice, in image-guided procedures, 114–15

lesion location, terms about, 190

liability issues, 167–68

lift (mastopexy)
  appearance on imaging, 27
  architectural distortion after, 85
  term use/definition, 192, 202

lift (mastopexy) (*cont.*)
Linver, M. N., 8, 32
lipomas, 132
lobular/lobular cancer
    asymmetry and, 83
    term use/definition, 182, 201
lucency, term use/definition, 188, 202
lump. *See* palpable abnormality
lumpectomy
    appearance on imaging, 26
    architectural distortion after, 85
    postlumpectomy/postradiation changes, 105*f*
    postoperative complication evaluation, 113
    term use/definition, 186, 192, 202
    ultrasound study after, 146*f*
lymph nodes
    benign evaluation/diagnoses of, 133
    bilateral abnormal axillary, 153*f*
    normal intramammary appearance, 133*f*
lymphoproliferative disorders, 153

magnetic resonance imaging. *See* MRI
    (magnetic resonance imaging)
male gynecomastia, 154*f*
male patients, 154–55
malignant/malignancy, term use/definition, 181,
    186, 202
mammogram
    breast anatomy view, 60*f*
    of breast density types, 58–59*f*
    reading/interpretation of, 60–62
    of retroareolar region, 95*f*
    showing density types, 174*f*
mammography. *See also* diagnostic
    mammogram; screening mammography;
    tomosynthesis (3-D mammography)
    as breast imaging test, 43–44
    in diagnostic evaluation, 66–67
    liability issues, 168
    mammogram image, 46*f*
    mortality rates and, 7, 56
    patient questions about, 159, 163
    risk-benefit ratio of, 169–70
    as screening tool, 56
    term use/definition, 183, 188, 202
Mammography Quality Standards Act.
    See MQSA (Mammography Quality
    Standards Act)
Mammoland, 6, 10

mantle field irradiation, personal history
    of, 63
mass, 188, 202. *See also* palpable abnormality
mastectomy
    appearance on imaging, 26–27
    postoperative complication evaluation, 113
    term use/definition, 187, 192, 202
mastitis, 95, 99, 100, 111–13, 126
mastopexy (lift)
    appearance on imaging, 27
    architectural distortion after, 85
    term use/definition, 192, 202
Mayo Clinic, 13
medicolegal issues, 167–68
metastasis
    risk of death and, 16
    term use/definition, 202
metastatic, term use/definition, 182
metastatic disease, 68, 109–10, 140, 182, 202
mildly suspicious finding, term use/definition,
    181, 202
moderately suspicious finding, term use/
    definition, 181, 203
modified radical mastectomy, term use/
    definition, 187, 203
molecular imaging, 48–49, 171
Morris, E. A., 7
mortality/mortality rates
    for breast cancer, 12
    mammography and, 7, 56
    term use/definition, 183, 203
MQSA (Mammography Quality Standards
    Act), 34, 36, 69–71, 73, 157, 173, 203
MRI (magnetic resonance imaging)
    anxiety and, 100
    as breast imaging test, 45–46
    in diagnostic evaluation, 66–67
    liability issues, 168
    MRI image, 47*f*
    risk-benefit ratio of, 171
    terms about, 189
    term use/definition, 184, 203
MRI-guided/MRI-guided needle biopsy
    procedure, 119–20, 119*f*
    term use/definition, 185, 203
multicentric/multicentric finding, term use/
    definition, 182, 203
multifocal/multifocal finding, term use/
    definition, 182, 203

needle biopsy. *See also* image-guided procedures
appearance on imaging, 26
core needle biopsy, 185
MRI-guided, 119–20, 119*f*
patient questions about, 161
sampling illustration, 48*f*
needle localization/bracketing, 142*f*
negative/negative result, 180, 193, 203. *See also*
false negative; true negative
Nightingale, Florence, 114
nipple discharge, diagnostic evaluation
of, 92–97
nipple inversion, 97. *See also* skin changes
nipple sparing mastectomy, term use/
definition, 204
nipple-to-lesion distance (NLD), term use/
definition, 190, 203–4
nodule, term use/definition, 188, 204
nurse navigator, education/functions of, 34

o'clock position, term use/definition, 190, 204
Osler, William, 139
ovarian history, personal history of, 63
overdiagnosis/overtreatment, 15–18

pain/swelling, diagnostic evaluation of, 91–92
palpable, term use/definition, 192, 204
palpable abnormality, 68, 70, 89, 91–92, 95
papillary cancer, 93, 122, 123*f*
papillomas, 93, 96, 122
parenchyma/parenchymal pattern, 7, 72–73, 82,
84–85, 87–88, 92, 98–99, 103
Parker, S. H., 7
past surgical history, terms about, 186–87
pathologist, term use/definition, 204
patient responsibilities
breast health history knowledge, 26–27
completing plan of action, 28
current status knowledge, 27–28
family history knowledge, 25–26
personality issues and, 30
quick list of, 30
retrieval of prior films, 23–25
scheduling, 28–30
seeing referring doctor, 27
patients. *See also* diagnostic evaluation scenarios
common questions of, 159–63
follow-up by, 157
response to diagnosis, 4

Patton, George S., 169
PEM (positron emission mammography), term
use/definition, 184, 204
percutaneous, term use/definition, 184, 204
perimenopausal period, 92
personal history, 63
personality issues, 30
personnel. *See* nurse navigator; radiologic
technologist (RT); radiologist
phyllodes tumors, 122, 123
physical examination of the breast, terms about, 192
physical findings, diagnostic evaluation of
change in breast size, 99–100
nipple discharge, 92–97
pain/swelling, 91–92
palpable abnormality, 89–91
skin changes, 97–99
Pisano, E. D., 7
plan of action, completion of, 28
plateau, term use/definition, 189, 204
poorly defined nodule/mass, diagnostic
evaluation of, 80–82
positive/positive result, term use/definition,
194, 204
positron emission mammography (PEM)
as molecular imaging, 48
risk-benefit ratio of, 171
positron emission tomography (PET), 108
postradiation changes, 47, 105*f*, 143
post-traumatic cysts, appearance of, 133*f*
pregnancy, 151–52
pre-pectoral, term use/definition, 192, 204
previous benign biopsy, 102–4
previous breast cancer/lumpectomy, 104–7
previous lesions, 100–102
primary tumor, search for, 109–10
prior radiation therapy, appearance on
imaging, 26
probably benign
surveillance of previous lesions, 100–102
term use/definition, 181, 204
procedures/biopsies, terms about, 184–86
prognosis, term use/definition, 204
progressive, term use/definition, 189
progressive enhancement, term use/
definition, 204

quadrant, term use/definition, 190, 204
questions, of patients, 159–63

radial scar, 85, 87, 122–23
radiation/radiation therapy
    calcifications and, 74
    in history of breast cancer, 104, 106
    history of chest irradiation and, 63
    imaging after surgery, 143–47
    in mammography, 7, 43, 159–60, 163, 169–70, 172, 183, 202
    in MRI/molecular imaging, 171
    overdiagnosis vs. overtreatment and, 15–16
    patient concerns/questions about, 99, 139
    in pregnancy, 151
    RT education on, 34
    skin thickening and, 26
radiography, term use/definition, 205
radiologic-pathologic correlation
    in image-guided procedures, 121–23
    term use/definition, 186, 205
radiologic technologist (RT)
    in breast imaging process, 55
    education/functions of, 34–35
    term use/definition, 194–95, 205
radiologist
    in diagnostic evaluation process, 66
    education/functions of, 32–33
    liability issues, 167–68
    referral-consult relationship, 38–40
    responsibilities of, 156–57
    term use/definition, 194, 205
radiology, role of
    on day of surgery, 141–43
    first imaging after surgery, 143–46
    imaging after treatment, 146
    in preoperative chemotherapy, 146–47
    provision of imaging data, 139
    when diagnosis is made, 140–41
radiology consult
    on active participation of patients, 31
    on annual screening, 19, 65
    on architectural distortion, 87
    on asymmetric density, 84
    on biopsy follow-up, 104
    on breast augmentation, 154
    on breast conservation therapy, 107
    on breast density, 178
    on breast imaging services/team, 35, 49
    on cancer diagnosis, 147
    on changes in breast size, 100
    on communication, 157–58

on cysts, 79
on early detection, 78
on image-guided procedures, 126
on incidental findings, 109
on inflammatory breast cancer, 113
on liability issues, 168
on mammography, 37, 172
on mastitis-type symptoms, 113
on menstrual cycles/breast tenderness, 74
on nipple discharge, 97
on palpable abnormality, 91
on patient questions, 163
for perimenopausal women, 92
on probably benign findings, 102
on radiologist/referring physician issues, 40
on range of breast conditions, 138
on screening/diagnostic evaluation process, 55
on skin changes, 98–99
on source/primary tumors, 110
on term meanings, 195
on ultrasound use, 82
randomized controlled trials (RCTs), 13–15
recall/callbacks
    for architectural distortion, 85–87
    for asymmetric density, 82–84
    for calcifications, 74–78
    in diagnostic evaluation, 71–73
    patient questions about, 162
    term use/definition, 205
    of well-defined nodules/masses, 78–82
reconstruction
    mammography screening following, 106
    term use/definition, 193, 205
reduction/reduction mammoplasty
    appearance on imaging, 27
    architectural distortion after, 85
    term use/definition, 192, 205
referring physicians
    patient responsibility to see, 27
    referral-consult relationship, 38–40
    responsibilities of, 157
refusal to consent for diagnostic procedure/ imaging, 29b
reporting categories. See BIRADS (Breast Imaging Reporting and Data System)
retraction, 97. See also skin changes
retroareolar/retroareolar region
    mammogram of, 95f
    term use/definition, 190, 205

retropectoral, term use/definition, 192, 205

risk-benefit ratio
  of mammography, 169–70
  of molecular imaging, 171
  of MRI, 171
  of sonography, 170

risk factors, for developing breast cancer, 18–19

Rockefeller, John D., 23

Rose, S. L., 8, 18

routine/routine image, term use/definition,
  187, 205

SBE (self breast examination)
  patient questions about, 160
  term use/definition, 192, 205

scattered, term use/definition, 190, 205

scheduling, patient responsibilities for, 28–30

screening mammography. *See also* diagnostic
    mammogram; mammography
  in advanced age, 64–65
  dense breast tissue and, 62
  diagnostic evaluation and, 3–7, 10
  for general population, 56–57
  guidelines controversy, 11–13
  for high-risk populations, 63–64
  overdiagnosis/overtreatment concerns, 15–18
  patient questions about, 162
  risk-based screening recommendations, 18–19
  RTCs and, 13–15
  tomosynthesis benefits, 18

screening patients, 53, 54*f*

sebaceous glands/cysts, 98, 133–34, 134*f*

secretory disease, 134

self breast examination (SBE)
  patient questions about, 160
  term use/definition, 192, 205

sensitivity, term use/definition, 194, 206

shadowing, term use/definition, 188–89, 206

short-interval follow-up, term use/definition,
  187, 206

Sickles, E. A., 8

simple mastectomy, term use/definition,
  187, 206

skin calcifications, 134

skin changes, diagnostic evaluation of, 97–99

skin lesions, 98, 134, 134*f*

skin-sparing mastectomy, term use/
    definition, 206

Smothers-Jones, B., 10

Society of Breast Imaging (SBI), 11–12, 37,
  56, 178

solid/solid lesion, term use/definition, 189, 206

solitary/solitary finding, term use/definition,
  190, 206

sonography. *See* ultrasound (sonography)

special cases
  breast implants, 152–53
  lactation/breastfeeding, 152
  lymphoproliferative disorders, 153
  male patients, 154–55
  pregnancy, 151–52

specificity
  of findings, 75
  term use/definition, 194, 206

statistics, terms about, 193–94

Stavros, A. T., 7

stereotactically guided
    (mammogram-guided) biopsy
  as image-guided procedure, 117–19, 117*f*
  term use/definition, 185, 206

subcutaneous mastectomy, term use/definition,
  187, 206

supplemental imaging, for high-risk patients, 64

surgical specimen, image of, 144*f*

surgical/surgical biopsy, term use/definition,
  185–86, 207

surveillance
  of previous lesions, 100–102
  term use/definition, 187, 207

survival rates, for breast cancer, 12

suspicious calcifications, 76*f. See also*
    calcifications

suspicious mass, characteristics of, 81*f*

suspicious/suspicious finding, term use/
    definition, 181, 207

swelling/pain, diagnostic evaluation of, 91–92

symptomatic patients, diagnostic evaluation of
  age criteria/guidelines, 67
  as anxiety-provoking, 66
  diagnostic symptoms, 68*b*
  indications for, 67–69
  of physical findings, 87–89
  recalls/callbacks, 71–73
  reporting categories, 69–71

synchronous, term use/definition, 182, 207

Tabár, L., 7, 15

technical recall, 72–73. *See also* recall/callbacks

terms
about breast surgeries for benign
conditions, 192
about breast tissue composition, 191
about breast ultrasound, 188–89
about cancer-related breast
surgeries, 192–93
about conclusions and recommendations, 191
about distribution of findings, 190–91, 192
about lesion location, 190
about personnel, 194–95
about physical examination of the
breast, 192
about statistics, 193–94
about understanding breast MRI, 189
Thatcher, Margaret, 11
thickening. *See* palpable abnormality
tomosynthesis (3-D mammography)
asymmetric density and, 84
benefits of, 18
breast density and, 62, 177
as breast imaging test, 44
illustration of, 46*f*
introduction of, 8
for poorly defined nodule/mass, 80
reading/interpretation of, 61
term use/definition, 183, 207
TRAM (transverse rectus abdominis
myocutaneous) flap, term use/definition,
193, 207
trauma areas, 133, 133*f*
true negative
as evaluation outcome, 127
term use/definition, 193, 207

true positive
as evaluation outcome, 127
term use/definition, 194, 207
tumor, term use/definition, 189, 207

ultrasound (sonography)
after lumpectomy, 146*f*
as breast imaging test, 45
in diagnostic evaluation, 66–67
free silicone on, 131, 131*f*
image of, 47*f*
of intraductal lesion, 96*f*
patient questions about, 159
for pregnant patients, 152
risk-benefit ratio of, 170
term use/definition, 183, 185, 188–89, 207–8
ultrasound-guided core biopsy, 115–16, 115*f*
unilateral
as cancer term, 182
term use/definition, 191, 208
urgency, in breast imaging, 111–13
U.S. Preventive Services Take Force (USPSTF),
11–15, 18–19, 38

valves, implant, 132*f*
vascular calcifications, 134–35, 135*f*

washout, term use/definition, 189, 208
well-defined nodules/masses
characteristic appearance of, 79*f*
recall/callbacks for, 78–82
Whitman, Walt, 151
whole-body PET scan, 108
workup, need for, 72